Free
to be Fit

BOB & YVONNE TURNBULL

Free to be Fit

BETHANY HOUSE PUBLISHERS
MINNEAPOLIS, MINNESOTA 55438
A Division of Bethany Fellowship, Inc.

ISBN 0-87123-165-4

Published by Bethany House Publishers
A Division of Bethany Fellowship, Inc.
6820 Auto Club Road, Minneapolis, Minnesota 55438

Printed in the United States of America

THE AUTHORS

BOB TURNBULL holds a Ph.D. in Psychology, and is an ordained Baptist minister. He is the Physical Fitness Specialist on the nationally syndicated early-morning "U. S. a.m." TV show, and the author of five previous books. For many years he was the internationally known "Chaplain of Waikiki Beach."

YVONNE TURNBULL recently won the Silver Angel, the "Oscar" of the religious world, for *The Living Cookbook.* She is the Home Nutritionist for the nationally syndicated "700 Club." She holds a B.S. degree in Psychology, and joins her husband in touring the nation presenting "Shape Up, America!" nutrition and physical fitness seminars.

A note to the reader:

Before you start any exercise program, we advise that you consult your physician. Only he/she can safely advise as to how much and what kind of exercise you should attempt.

CONTENTS

PHOTO LIST

FOREWORD

I have known Bob and Yvonne Turnbull for the past several years. They truly live their Christian faith, not only spiritually and mentally, but physically.

Bob is the Physical Fitness Specialist for our "U.S. a.m." nationally syndicated TV show; and Yvonne, for the past three years, has been the Nutritionist on "The 700 Club," another of our national television shows. The response by our viewing public to their godly health tips has been tremendous.

The scriptural theme for *Free To Be Fit* is based on 1 Corinthians 6:19 and 20; 10:31. Bob and Yvonne believe our Lord came to minister to "the whole person." Many Christians are maturing well in the spiritual and mental realm but neglectful of their bodies. The purpose of this book is to shore up that void and present simple, workable procedures for becoming healthier, following guidelines from the Bible and nature.

Free To Be Fit will show you *why* you should exercise regularly and *how* to do it. They will show you how to once-and-for-all take off and keep off excess weight. The book also presents a simple, delicious and nutritious eating plan for the entire family.

If you apply the principles of *Free To Be Fit,* your health will immediately improve and you will have more energy and vitality for God's service.

This book can improve and change your life!

Pat Robertson
President
Christian Broadcasting
Network

ACKNOWLEDGMENTS

We wish to thank the following people for their kind assistance in putting together *Free To Be Fit*:

Pat Robertson and Tommy John for their warm endorsements;

Doug Bethune for his fine photographs—both on the cover and on the inside;

Robert Stone and Olaf John for their help with the manuscript.

INTRODUCTION

Bob Turnbull is one of my best friends in sports ministries. When Bob was the "Chaplain of Waikiki Beach" and my wife, Sally, and I occasionally visited Honolulu, we would also give Bob a call—we often sat and talked for hours about our lives, physical and spiritual; we also enjoyed some plain old baseball shoptalk!

I am very happy that Bob and Yvonne have written *Free To Be Fit*. They have always impressed me as being physically fit, and I know that they are *spiritually* fit, too. I once heard Bob give the L. A. Dodgers a chapel talk, and he really hit home (if you'll pardon the pun) in terms a baseball player could understand and identify with.

You don't have to play professional baseball to need physical fitness. Bob and Yvonne have written a practical and helpful book for those of you who would rather watch than play the game!

Tommy John
California Angels

Chapter One

EXERCISE AS A GIFT TO YOURSELF

If you lived in the right part of Southern California and got up early enough in the morning, you might see a trim, athletic woman with flowing, silvery hair, heading out for a morning run. Then if you waited you would see her dive into an Olympic-size swimming pool to swim a vigorous sixteen laps.

This woman is 71 years old. She is Bob's mother, Dr. Amorita Treganza—not a lifelong athlete, but a woman who has known the pressures of both motherhood and business. At age 60 she saw herself slipping into an easy acceptance of more weight, less energy and less strength. She decided to change the direction of her life by changing the direction of her aging. Gradually she changed her diet toward natural foods and developed a program of regular exercise.

This woman had discovered that she had been accepting a gradual, but unnecessary, deterioration of her body. She decided to reverse this process. And she did. After a slow and cautious start, she began to experience new energy, a new suppleness and a better attitude toward living a complicated professional life; she now possesses new vitality, within and without. Her decision to change soon showed all over. She was no longer a sluggish victim of sedentary life.

What are some of the effects of the sedentary life? What are some of the symptoms which we so easily accept as necessary, inevitable and irreversible results of growing older? Here are some that are easy to spot:

Reduced energy
Anxiety felt as tension, depression, irritability, sleeplessness
Dizziness, lightheadedness, a palpitating or fluttering heart
Shortness of breath
Indigestion, heartburn, gas, belching, stomach cramps,
   irregularity
Stiffness in the joints and bones
Cold hands or cold feet
Back or shoulder pain

All of these are symptoms of *advanced* age and/or of the sedentary life. If you are under age 75, however, there is no excuse for these symptoms to be a regular part of your life. Even if you are over 75, these symptoms can be significantly reduced by proper exercise and nutrition.

Among Americans, many of these signs of advanced age begin to show up before a person is middle-aged. Studies show that for average Americans blood flow from the heart decreases 40% by age 25. In other words, the heart is working 40% less effectively than it ought to be working. By age 35 that reduction often reaches 60%! The "good life" of comfort and ease enjoyed by many Americans is also accompanied by loss of energy, shortness of breath, lightheadedness, stomach problems, aches and pains. And all these occur because of a lack of exercise.

The key to vital physical health is *blood circulation*. And the key to blood circulation is exercise. That major muscle of life, the heart, pumps blood to every area of the body. If the heart becomes sluggish, weak or lazy, it simply does not push as much blood to the extremities of the body. The results have already been listed.

Research has repeatedly shown that as the heart is exercised, it becomes a distinctly more efficient instrument, capable of doing more while working less. In the properly exercised heart, the muscle fibers of the heart are lengthened. This lengthening of the fibers allows the heart chambers to pump more blood with each contraction. Resultantly, the arteries serving the heart enlarge. Larger arteries carry more blood, and more blood means a greater supply of oxygen to the parts of the body. Researchers at the University of Minnesota recently discovered that the blood flow from a well-exercised heart may be as much as five times that of the blood flow from a sedentary heart.

Exercise helps the heart to pump more blood with each beat. The healthy, active heart therefore pumps more blood with fewer beats, and does not need to beat as frequently. It is common among people who exercise to find that their resting heart rate has decreased ten to twenty beats since they began their exercise program.

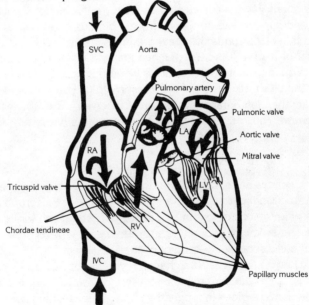

Just like any other muscle, the heart increases in strength and efficiency when subjected to regular exercise.

But most Americans' hearts are in terrible shape. Too much eating, too much drinking, too much weight, and too little exercise all contribute to a weakened heart. Thomas J. Bassler, a California pathologist, says that, on the basis of the thousands of autopsies he has performed, he concludes that two out of every three adult deaths are premature. These deaths are related to what he calls "the loafer's heart."

Thomas K. Cureton, a professor at the University of Illinois Physical Fitness Laboratory, says, "The average American young man has a middle-aged body. He can't run the length of a city block; he can't climb a flight of stairs without getting breathless. In his twenties he has the capacity that a man is expected to have in his forties."

Cureton goes on to say, "The average middle-aged man in this country is close to death. He is only one emotional shock or one sudden exertion away from a serious heart attack." If you think Cureton is overstating the case, start looking at the ages of people listed in your newspaper's obituary column.

You're probably beginning to wonder if *your* body is "older" than it should be and if there is something you can do to reverse the deterioration that you've allowed. The answer is *change*. You must now begin to *change* the way you live.

Modifying Your Behavior Toward More Activity

Chances are good that you will not be able to change your way of living overnight. Even if you hit the road tomorrow morning for a bit of jogging, by the next morning you will be so stiff and sore that you will need three days to recover. You will become discouraged and soon give up.

But you can set about changing your life-style *slowly*. You can adopt a pattern of regular activity. Don't wait for something sudden and serious to trigger the change—something like bad news from your physician. Begin now to slowly modify your style of life. It may be helpful to start by simply *altering your thinking*.

We met Paul Bragg on the beach at Waikiki. He was in his nineties at the time, but a living exponent of exercise and healthy living. Paul led exercise classes daily for people on the beach. He coralled the fat, the flabby, the sluggish and the lazy wherever he found them, and got them to join him for exercises on the beach. He scolded them, he prodded them, he tempted them. He did everything he could to get them to exercise. And once they started, they never stopped. They felt the difference, saw the difference and enjoyed the difference!

As a central part of his routine, Paul repeated the following positive phrases:

My mind is the master of my body.

I choose to direct my living with intelligence, knowledge and wisdom.

I see myself exercising, eating properly and acquiring healthful living habits.

I have the power given by my Creator to direct my body to do what I command.

I no longer want to walk the dead-end road I am presently walking. Instead, I choose to live a healthy, wholesome, long, active, productive life.

This may be how you can begin. Read these statements again. Now read them aloud and with conviction.

Now, stand up. Put your feet apart and raise your hands as high as you can toward the ceiling. Then stretch, turn, reach, inhale deeply, and then exhale.

You have already begun to change. You have done something different. You have modified your behavior. You have begun to take control of your body!

Before this day is over, do something physically active. Take a fifteen-minute walk; or play a game of badminton; or throw a frisbee; or shoot a few baskets; or spend five minutes bending, stretching and moving your body. Do it to seal this bargain you just made with yourself. Do it as a celebration of a joyous event. You are giving a gift to yourself—the gift of vibrant health.

Then, as soon as you have a chance, tell someone you

know and trust about what you have committed yourself to do for yourself. If you have a co-worker, a Christian friend or another household member who might have an interest in what you are deciding to do, tell him or her. And invite that person to join you.

And we encourage you as John encouraged his fellow-believers during the first century: "Beloved, I pray that in all respects you may prosper and be in good health, just as your soul prospers" (3 John 2, NASB).

Chapter Two

A NEW ATTITUDE ABOUT YOURSELF

Many people are dismayed by the very thought of physical exercise. Exercise, they think, causes only pain. And they are especially uncomfortable about the fact that most exercise is so *visible*. Almost always it's public. To exercise they must often go to places where other people can see them.

A person who is self-consciously out of shape can think of nothing worse than public exercise—especially if that person is overweight. The fat person imagines himself out on the street in a pair of old-fashioned boxer shorts, belly bouncing up and down, legs chafed raw—with all the neighbors snickering.

But three things may help to overcome this uncomfortable image about exercise. The first is to *think* about yourself differently and let your mind provide a different picture of things. For example, if you're feeling "up tight," imagine yourself standing on a magnificent beach, the water flowing over your feet, the sun bathing your skin. You feel vigorous, warm, secure.

Then imagine looking across the bright blue water to where the sun is playing upon the waves, turning the water silver. Now notice your emotions. You are relaxed. You are enjoying the "mood" you have created. And though it is only a mental picture, your body is sharing the experience. There is an immense amount of pleasure which your mind can generate all by itself for you. You can actually change your feelings about things by changing your thinking about those things.

You need to think differently about yourself, about your body. Decide to agree with the Scriptures: "For thou didst form my inward parts: Thou didst weave me in my mother's womb. I will give thanks to Thee, for I am fearfully and wonderfully made" (Ps. 139:13, 14, NASB). As you change your thinking about your body, you can begin to think differently about bodily movement. Movement makes you aware of the environment in which you live. By moving you experience your environment. Increased awareness of the environment means increased sensitivity. And increased sensitivity brings a stronger sense of the vitality and strength contained in your own body. You, all by yourself, can generate a sense of personal endurance, strength and power.

Some psychologists insist that both obesity and its accompanying sense of weakness and inferiority are produced by an unconscious hatred of one's body. What we wish to propose here, however, is a change in your attitude toward your body. You can learn to like yourself, to respect yourself, to rejoice in the strength and vitality of your body. You can learn to rejoice in the fact that, indeed, you *are* fearfully and wonderfully made.

A second thing which can change the negative image of exercise is *activity* itself. Getting active is really quite simple. Here are a few suggestions:

Take a five-minute walk during your lunch break. As you walk, watch children playing in a park or observe the pedestrian traffic in your downtown area.

Park a block away from the store next time you go shopping. Walk the rest of the way.

Get up early in the morning, get dressed and take a short walk around the yard or through the neighborhood.

Instead of watching television after dinner, take a walk around the block. Choose never to miss a sunset again if you can help it.

Use the stairway instead of the elevator in a building that offers a choice. Start by walking up just one flight, then taking the elevator at the second floor. Take more stairs as your fitness improves.

Stand when you would normally look for a place to sit.

Anticipate situations in which you can *use* your body instead of some mechanical substitute.

None of these suggestions require a strenuous exercise plan. But if you combine just a few of them, you will acquire a new sense of both your body and the environment in which it moves. You may even become aware of sights and smells and sounds which are new to you. They were always there, but you had shut them out, ignored them, passed them by. Once you become aware of the powers of perception which reside in your body, you are well on the way to a new sensitivity, a new enjoyment of your body.

A third thing you can do is to relieve some of the tensions, experienced in work or other responsibilities of life, by using some simple exercises that can be done nearly anywhere. They are very useful, because they relieve tension caused by nervousness, emotional strain or concentrated thought.

These exercises stretch, tone and release tension all at the same time.

Here are a few simple exercises which you should be able to adapt to various situations and settings.

Have you been sitting at a desk for a couple of hours? Feel tense? As in the photograph below, place your hands on the front corners of your chair, then lift your knees as close to your face as possible. Hold this position for a few seconds.

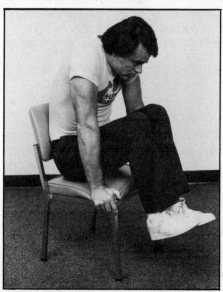

Here's another simple exercise. Sit erect in your chair. Now lean forward and reach for your ankles with both hands, keeping both legs straight. Move your head down toward your knees. If you can touch your knees with your forehead, good. Do it once more. If you feel pain, stop.

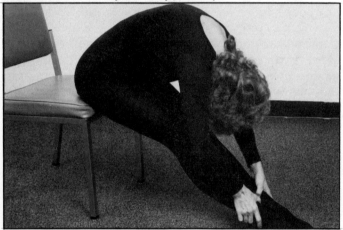

Sit up straight once again. Hold your arms over your head, with fingers interlocked, and stretch toward the ceiling. Now return to your normal sitting position.

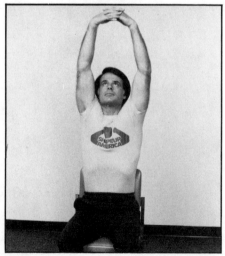

Chapter Three

AEROBICS FOR A LONGER LIFE

You now are ready at least to *think* about a program of exercise. The big word today in exercise is "aerobics." Aerobics, briefly, is steady exercise which demands an uninterrupted exertion from your muscles for a minimum of 12 minutes, preferably longer.

The word aerobic actually means air, but more specifically it refers to the oxygen in the air. Muscles need oxygen to function, and their need for oxygen increases dramatically when they are worked. How hard a muscle is working can be measured by how much oxygen it uses (burns). The harder the exercise, the greater the amount of oxygen required; the greater the amount of oxygen required, the faster the heart must beat.

If a person makes a muscle work too hard, its demand for oxygen will be greater than the heart can deliver. Aerobic exercises are designed to make the muscles work hard enough to require lots of oxygen but not so hard as to exceed the ability of the heart to pump freshly oxygenated blood to it. Aerobic exercises, according to Dr. Kenneth Cooper, are "a variety of exercises that stimulate heart and lung activity for a time period sufficiently long to produce beneficial changes in the body."

Activity that uses muscles could be called exercise. And any exercise helps to tone muscles. But to derive the greatest benefit for a muscle from a particular exercise or movement requires some strategy. The shortest exercise of greatest benefit for a muscle is what an exercise program should achieve. This is aerobics' forte. Fifteen minutes of jogging, for example,

25

may provide as much benefit as two hours of tennis or four hours of housecleaning. And aerobics is one of the fastest ways to decrease body fat. This includes not only noticeable fat, such as the roll around the middle, but fat within the muscles which can be replaced with solid muscle.

The main criterion for exercise is that it provide movement for bones and muscle. But there are *three* criteria for aerobic exercise: continuous, steady, intense. This means that many "traditional" exercises really are not aerobic. The chart below lists various exercises. Some are aerobic; some are nonaerobic.

Aerobic	*Nonaerobic*
Fast walking	Tennis
Running/Jogging	Downhill skiing
Cross-country skiing	Football
Jumping rope	Calisthenics
Running in place	Racquetball
Bicycling	Weight lifting
Stationary cycling	Square dancing
Rowing	Bowling
Mini-trampoline (Rebounder)	Canasta
Swimming	Volleyball

You may be surprised to see what is included among the nonaerobic exercises. Canasta and Racquetball do not seem to be at all similar forms of exercise. But they are both nonaerobic. The reason is that racquetball is a stop-and-go sport (not continuous/steady). It requires quick spurts of activity, but not continuous activity. Canasta, a card game, has little intensity, though it may require some steady effort.

Your Training Rate

When starting your aerobics program, you may ask, "How hard should I exercise?" This is a very important question. Your pulse rate is the indicator; it will tell you how hard you can exercise. It will also protect you from overexertion. During an aerobic exercise you will want to raise your pulse rate to 70%-85% of your maximum heart rate, and keep it there for at least 12 minutes without stopping. This will be your "training rate."

Your training rate is calculated by first figuring your maximum heart rate. The maximum rate at which a human heart can beat is 220 beats per minute, but this decreases in adulthood. To figure your maximum heart rate, subtract your age from 220. For example, if you are 35 years old, your maximum pulse rate would be 185 (220-35=185).

Your training rate will be 70%-85% of your maximum heart rate. Therefore, if you are 35 your training rate would be between 130 and 157.

If you have not exercised for a long time or if you are overweight, you should begin exercising at 60% of your maximum heart rate, and then gradually work your way up to 70%-85%. (Training at below 70% will not produce much improvement. Training at above 85% can be harmful.) If you have a history of heart disease, it is recommended that you do not exercise at over 75% of your maximum heart rate.

After you have completed your aerobic exercise, you should immediately take your pulse rate (PR) to see if you were exercising within your training rate. When you are beginning your program, it is also good to stop momentarily during the exercise and take your pulse. This will help you judge if you are going too slow or too fast (by seeing if your heart rate is too low or too high). After doing this a few times you will know, without stopping, at what pace you should be exercising.

By monitoring your pulse rate you are exercising at your own rate and not at someone else's. For instance, some people who are really out of shape could zoom their pulse rate up to their training rate by just going on a slow walk, whereas someone else might have to go on a fast run to achieve the same effect.

Some exercises will take a few minutes to get your heart rate up to its training rate. Running is a good example. After stretching and loosening up, you should walk fast, then jog, then run. Therefore, your heart doesn't reach its training rate immediately. Because of this, you must run for 15 to 18 minutes, thus allowing three minutes for the pulse to reach its correct level.

Training Rates

Age	Maximum heart rate	Training rates
20	200	140-170
25	195	137-165
30	190	133-162
35	185	130-157
40	180	126-153
45	175	123-149
50	170	119-145
55	165	116-140
60	160	112-136
65	155	109-132

Your Recovery Heart Rate

Your heart should return to its normal rate in a short period of time after completion of an exercise. Dr. Cooper, who pioneered aerobics research, claims that the *recovery* heart rate gives the best indication of how much exercise you can safely handle. Your recovery heart rate is measured *after* you have exercised. Five minutes after you have stopped, your pulse rate should be below 120. Ten minutes after you have stopped, your pulse rate should have dropped down below 100. If your recovery heart rate is higher than these figures, you should assume that your routine was too vigorous.

How to Take Your Pulse

You will need a watch with a sweep second hand, or a stopwatch for this.

Place your first two fingers on either the inside wrist or the neck area beside the "Adam's apple." Do not use your thumb—it has a pulse of its own. Press just hard enough so that you can feel the rhythmic beat.

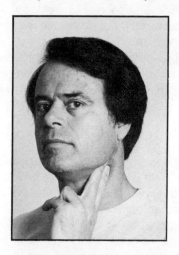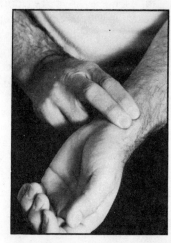

Count the beats for six seconds, then multiply that number by ten. The reason you should not count for 60, 15, or even 10 seconds is that there is a greater chance of taking an inaccurate count. Also, your heart rate slows down very quickly once you stop exercising, so you will have less chance of taking a correct reading.

A resting pulse rate for most men is from 72-76, and for most women, from 75-82.

Examples of Aerobic Exercises

Walking

When you were a kid, you probably did a great deal of walking. But as you got older it became "uncool," so you started driving all the time. And since most people need to get some place in a hurry, there was no time for walking—gotta grab the wheels and zip!

Walking can increase your pulse rate if you walk *briskly*. No easy strolling. The latter is fine on the proverbial moon-lit night, but not if you want an effective aerobic exercise. A brisk walk is easier on your joints and knees than jogging or running, especially if you're pounding on concrete or blacktop.

Just as with any of the exercises, start out slowly and work up to a vigorous pace. Keep it there from 12 to 15 minutes (or longer if you wish). Cool down by slowing your pace for a couple of minutes. Don't forget to use a very good pair of walking shoes. Your feet must be well-supported.

Bicycling

You can either go biking outside or you can pump the pedals indoors on a stationary bike. Both give you the same benefits as long as you work to get the pulse rate up. The gears of your bike will help you when you go uphill so you won't push your heart rate above what it should be.

When biking indoors you can watch TV, study your Bible, listen to recordings, or read. You obviously need your legs for this one, but your arms are free to make this exercise a two-in-one activity.

There are many stationary bicycles to choose from, ranging in price from $70 to $1,000. You can purchase a good bike for around $100. Stay away from the motor-driven bikes. They do all the work for you and that would be self-defeating. When purchasing a bike, look for one that has a comfortable seat, an adjustable resistance on the wheel and a light but solid frame. If you want to strengthen your thighs, tighten the tension! If you want to slim them down, loosen the tension and pedal faster.

Aerobic Dancing or Calisthenics

If you enjoy music, you will enjoy exercising aerobically by doing calisthenics or dance movements. Just make sure you stretch first (see chapter four). Women especially are participating in this popular type of exercise. However, this form of exercise isn't exclusively for the *fairer* sex. It is for both sexes and all ages. Because of our cultural mores, very few men will perform a combination of aerobic dancing and calisthenics to music, especially if being observed by several women. But if they would, they would reap many positive benefits. Whether you perform this exercise—often called dancercise, jazzercise or praisercise—at home, at the Y or at a spa, you will certainly feel you've had a good workout—and you have!

Swimming

If you have lower back problems, swimming is an excellent choice. And this is a terrific exercise for the whole body because it works all of your muscle groups.

To derive the maximum benefit, swim for *time*, rather than for speed or distance. However, you can't just float around and occasionally paddle. You can do any type of stroke you prefer, but make sure you swim continuously for a minimum of 12 minutes with your heart pumping at its training rate. Otherwise you won't realize cardiovascular benefits. But just like any exercise, begin slowly and build up gradually.

If, however, you are looking to lose body fat, this is not the best exercise to do. Tests at Dr. Kenneth Cooper's clinic in Dallas have shown that there will not be a great reduction in body fat, for in water the body tends to conserve its fat to provide warmth and buoyancy. But even though it won't reduce the fat, neither will it add any to your body.

One good test to see if you have a lot of fat on your body is to float. Fat floats easily.

Running and Jogging*

Running and jogging are the best known forms of aerobic exercise. It has been shown that you will get the fastest fat loss using either of these two exercises.

---

*See Appendix for further information.

What distinguishes a jogger from a runner usually has to do with the amount of time it takes a person to run a mile. If you can finish a mile in eight minutes or less, you are a runner. A jogger, however, is someone who doesn't care how long he takes to run a mile, so he generally takes more than eight minutes. But while the clock is used to make the distinction, the *attitude* is really what counts; we've known *marathon* runners who must be classified technically as joggers, since their only real concern is to stay ahead of the small truck bearing a sign saying, "End of Race. Resume Normal traffic."

Jogging reaps tremendous rewards for the body. When we lived in Honolulu, a friend of ours named Judy decided she was going to run a marathon which is held every December in Honolulu. So she started training. Slowly. Over a period of time she increased her running ability, kept losing fat and wound up looking delightfully slim in a matter of months. When she ran the marathon that December, she looked great and felt great.

Many women feel apprehensive about running outdoors, especially if they're overweight. And, of course, due to today's moral decay, it's not always safe for a woman to run, especially along certain public streets and at specific times of the early morning or late evening. Some women tell us they run *and* pray in certain locations! A friend of ours in Los Angeles says, "I never have any problems with my jogging at night—not with my two Dobermans running with me!" No argument there! If there's any chance of foul play, *don't run alone.*

Why not set up a jogging course in your own home if you don't want to gallop outside? Start in the kitchen, then jog into your living room, around to the bedroom and back again. It's all right to run in circles, so to speak. You probably do it, sometimes, in other areas of your life, don't you? Keep track of your time and your pulse rate.

We do this frequently when we travel. We will run inside our motel room, combining the running with some jump rope routines and calisthenics for a good workout.

Lest you become too discouraged at this point about running, we hasten to add that not everybody is geared mentally, psychologically or physically for running. Don't feel *guilty* if you do not want to jog or run. Walking is an excellent alternative; another that we enjoy is the rebounder (mini-trampoline).

Rebounding to Muscular Strength and Physical Fitness

Both of us love to run—on our mini-trampoline. It provides a very different feeling, buoyant, exhilarating. And we can accomplish in *12 minutes* what it used to take 40 minutes to accomplish running outside. During her first month-and-a-half of running on the rebounder, Yvonne lost inches off her hips, thighs and buttocks—inches that did not seem to budge during street running.

It is great fun to jump and run on the mini-trampoline. Anybody not physically impaired can do it. You can twist as you jump. You can kick your legs. You can even bounce on it while sitting down. The rebounder is great family fun for all ages. Even the ones least inclined to join you in a physical fitness program will not be able to resist the rebounder. And all this can be done *with* another activity, such as TV watching, record-listening, and even prayer and meditation. Running and jumping on the rebounder is one of the easiest of all the aerobics, and is our personal favorite.

Rebounding is also one of the most productive exercises because of the effect it has on circulation of the fluid around our cells called intercellular fluid. There is three times more of this fluid than blood in the body. Intercellular fluid is the cells' environment. It brings nutrients and carries away waste. It is like a second circulation system. This fluid flows through a system of valves, but these valves have no heart to force liquid through them. Instead, they are activated by changes of pressure caused by (1) muscular flexing and relaxing, and (2) changes in gravitational pull.

Vigorous muscular exercise, including the other aerobics just named, will cause an increase in circulation of intercellular fluid. Rebounding has been found to provide the greatest changes in pressure with the least muscular effort, because when you jump, your body changes velocity and direction twice. In one full bounce, you go from double the force of gravity to zero gravity. The vertical motion closes and opens the valves decisively, creating a squeezing of toxins which moves them out of the body quickly.

A woman we know who was in her mid-sixties, and was a semi-invalid, was given a rebounder by her health-minded son and daughter-in-law. The woman could not even stand comfortably on it, much less move her ankles to bounce. They showed her how to sit on it and bounce. She enjoyed that and did it a few minutes each day. After several days she was able to stand on it and bounce gently for three or four minutes. She gradually increased her bouncing to a jog, then to a run, then to a full-fledged aerobic exercise—over a period of three months. The last we heard was that she is gardening outside and needing to sleep only at night, whereas before she spent her days in bed and had been hardly able to complete household chores!

Exercising on the Rebounder

1. Before you start jumping or running on the rebounder, you must properly stretch.

2. Begin to bounce and jog lightly on the rebounder to warm up the muscles and enlarge the arteries, preparing the body for more vigorous exercise.

3. Run on the rebounder, knees up at least to your waist. Swing your arms naturally and freely, and breathe deeply. Continue non-stop for at least 12 to 15 minutes. (If you are just starting a rebounder program and can go only 4 to 5 minutes, don't strain yourself. If you do this six days a week, you will increase your running ability until you can go 12, 15, even 30 minutes. Just stay with it.)

4. Begin to "cool down" in order to bring your heart,

blood pressure and muscle activity into a recovery state. Decrease your run to a jog, then to a slow, light bounce. Do this for 2 to 3 minutes.

5. Finish with some calisthenics and stretching exercises. An obvious advantage of the rebounder is that its springy fabric surface does not cause the stress to joints that hard pavement causes. On the other hand, if you exercise on a rebounder, you don't "go" anywhere; you stay in one spot. So, if you're a sight-seer or a "fresh-air freak," you may prefer to walk, jog or run outdoors.

"...let us also lay aside every weight, and sin which clings so closely, and let us run with perseverance the race that is set before us, looking to Jesus the pioneer and perfecter of our faith..." (Heb. 12:1, 2a, RSV).

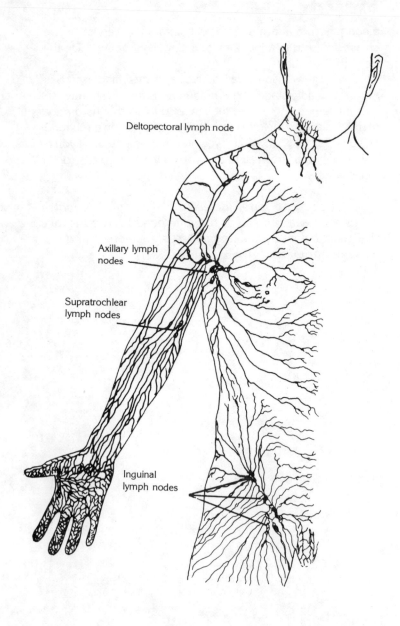

Deltopectoral lymph node

Axillary lymph nodes

Supratrochlear lymph nodes

Inguinal lymph nodes

Chapter Four

GAINING NEW STRENGTH WITH EXERCISE

Not long ago a friend named John told us of his recent purchase of a health club membership. For $300 a year he has access to the spa, including a ping-pong table, a chinning bar, a stationary bicycle, a steam room/sauna, a swimming pool and a weight-lifting machine. John has joined thousands of men and women of all ages who pour millions of dollars into health club bank accounts in hope of improving their health.

Unfortunately, health club memberships don't improve health—not much anyway. They may help people to do a few more push-ups, lift heavier weights, ride a bicycle longer, and hold out the hope of someday looking like an Atlas or a beach bunny. But the average club member doesn't ever do enough swimming, bicycle riding or anything else to improve his fitness.

In fact, a little investigation showed that the instructors and managers of John's club had not been trained in physical education or exercise physiology. They were principally salespeople, whose function was to sell memberships and equipment. Poor John admitted that not only had he bought a membership, but he had been convinced to make a down payment on a $700 treadmill which he could install in his basement.

Recently the American Medical Association Committee on Exercise issued a formal statement, calling into question the practices of many health club and exercise machine promoters—"Their most serious shortcoming is that most of them do little to improve fitness of the heart and lungs, which

are most in need of exercise today.... Real physical fitness results only with regular *overloads* (in intensity and duration) of
physical activity."

But lest you think that every health club operator is a huck-
ster, be assured that there are many top-notch health clubs out
there, and for the right person, a membership can be very
beneficial. A health club can provide equipment, encourage-
ment, and surroundings conducive both to a necessary "overload" in exercise and the relaxation which should follow. Not
many people can afford to buy for themselves sauna equipment, whirlpool facilities, universal weight-lifting machines,
dumbbells, a swimming pool, and treadmills. Thus, a club
membership *may* be a sound investment.

If you're determined to shell out money to use a commercial exercise facility, shop carefully and compare. Here are
some suggestions:

* Check with your Better Business Bureau. Find out what
  kind of laws exist in your state to regulate such establish-
  ments. And find out which clubs have a clean record.
* What does the club offer for facilities and equipment?
  Will you be able to perform a full variety of aerobic and
  nonaerobic exercises?
* Is the facility clean and well-maintained?
* Are the staff members well-trained and experienced? Or
  do they just happen to look good in a running suit?
* Is the schedule of the facility compatible with yours? If
  you're a woman, and can run only on Mondays, Wednes-
  days and Fridays, you'll be wasting your money if two of
  those days are for men only.

In this chapter we want to show you how to become a bit
stronger and a bit firmer by means of exercise. You don't need
a health club membership for these exercises; you can do
them at home. And if you are faithful, you will see dramatic results.

Quite often, people get confused by all of the terminology
associated with exercise physiology. There are calisthenics,

isometrics, isotonics, weight lifting, isokinetics, body-building, etc. Although you won't need the fancy terms to do the exercises, we'll give you a quick overview of some of the exercise jargon.

An *isometric* is a muscle-strengthening exercise in which a muscle fiber is shortened or constricted and held in such a position for a period of time. It is also called a muscle-resisting exercise. A group of muscles is contracted against another muscle or group of muscles, or against an immovable object. These exercises build strength. But isometrics do little to aid the cardiovascular system or to build endurance. However, isometrics can be practiced every day and almost anywhere. And many of them are convenient for people who otherwise keep very busy and don't easily find time to run or swim or play a sport.

An *isotonic* exercise is an exercise in which the body works against its own weight or against supplemental weights. Calisthenics and weight lifting are examples of isotonic exercises. Calisthenics are a set of rhythmic movements that develop both flexibility and strength.

Weight lifting will increase the size of muscles as well as build strength. The principle involved is simple: specific muscles are flexed against a strong opposing force—a weight. Pitting your muscles against weights to push, pull or lift, gradually builds strength in those muscles used. The muscles grow both in size and strength. For maximum growth and strength achievement, weight exercises should be done *every other day*, not every day.

An *isokinetic* exercise is also a resistance exercise. It combines principles of both isometric and isotonic exercise. Equipment which controls the amount of resistance, relative to the degree of exertion, is used for these exercises. Use of a "bullworker" (stretch cable) is an example of isokinetic exercise.

Following are some basic calisthenic exercises to practice. Do them anywhere from three to six days a week. You will be rewarded in a short time by a new sense of strength and suppleness. These are the exercises you should use before performing your regular aerobics.

Exercise in Action

Waist

Keep a weight (a book or a light dumbbell) nearby. Using the weight will provide added resistance and you'll get results more quickly.

1. Hold the weight in your right hand and press your left hand against the back of your head. Now bend to the right as far

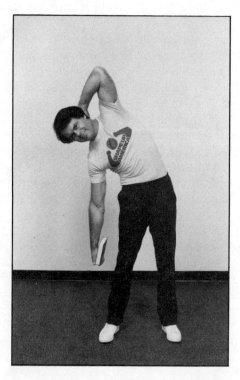

as you can go, bending from the waist. Try to keep your lower body stationary. Return to a standing position. Repeat at least 10 times. Do the same thing for your left side. Keep the hips stationary.

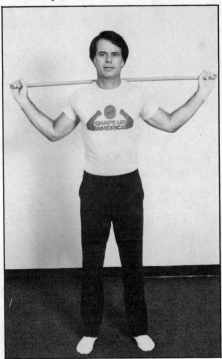

2. Take a light pole (e.g., a broom handle) and place it behind your head, resting it on your shoulders. Grab each end with a hand. Keeping your legs and hips pointing straight ahead, twist from the waist as far as you can turn to your left. Return to starting position and now twist to the right as far as you can. Repeat until you feel a "burning" feeling in your waist.

This "burn" occurs when you have worked a muscle strenuously. You will feel as if you cannot contract that muscle for another moment. Usually if you will take a breather for a few

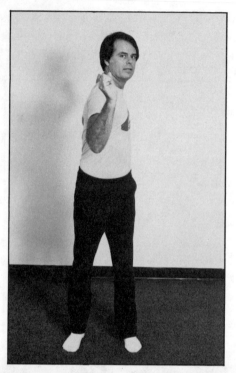

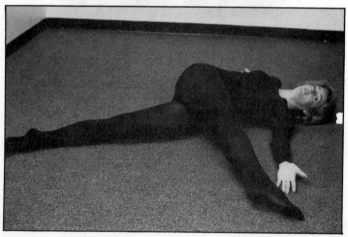

seconds, you can go back to that exercise. As you become more physically fit you will be able to exercise longer without experiencing the burn. The burn is caused by a lack of oxygen in the muscle, which allows a build-up of lactic acid. Better fitness will result in a greater volume of oxygen.

3. Lie flat on the floor with feet spread apart 12 inches and your arms outstretched to the side. Swing your right foot up and over and touch your left hand. Keep your left leg straight. Return to original position. Do the same with your left foot swinging over to touch your right hand.

Abdominals

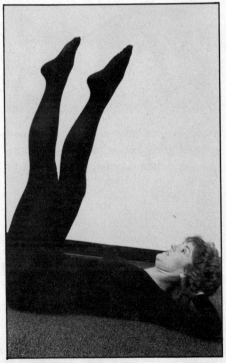

1. Lie on your back. Extend your legs straight up in the air.

Place your hands behind your head. Lift your head up. Cross your left leg over the right leg. Then cross your right leg over the left one. Do this in a rapid scissoring motion 10 to 15 times. Use your abdominal muscles to hold your head up—don't rely on your arms.

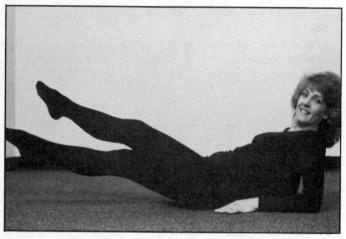

2. An advanced version of the first exercise would be to elevate yourself to rest on your elbows, palms flat on the floor. Scissor kick again, holding your legs just a few inches off the floor. Do this for 15 to 20 repetitions. Your tummy will certainly feel this one.

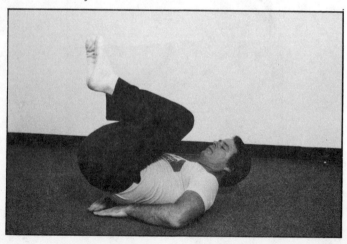

3. The basic sit-up is best done with your knees bent. Lie flat on the floor, hands behind your head, and bring yourself up to your knees and touch them with your elbows. Return to the floor. Repeat as many as you can, up to 50.

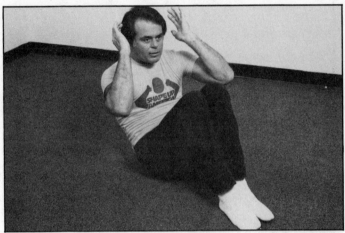

4. Here's a simple abdominal exercise that will have your mid-section quivering. Lie on the floor, with your head elevated just a bit and your arms at your side. Put your legs together, then elevate them just a few inches off the floor and hold them still for as long as you can. They'll drop sooner than you think. Your goal will be to hold this position for two minutes.

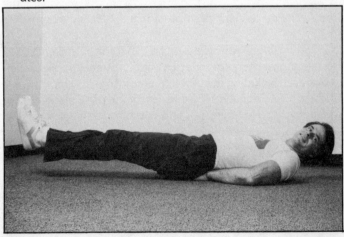

5. From the same position, place your hands near your buttocks, palms down. With your legs together on the floor, bring them up and try to touch your knees to your chest. Return them to the floor, slowly. Do 10 to 12 repetitions.

Legs, Hips and Thighs

Probably someone is now saying, "Oh, good! Now we can get into *spot reducing.*" Well, pause a moment, because here's a short sermon about spot reducing.

When we talk about spot reducing, we usually find women wanting to reduce their buttocks, hips and thighs, and men wanting to lose their overhanging bellies (so they won't get harpooned at the beach in the summer). Fair enough. But what do most people do? They try "gadgets." They wear "reducing" belts and rubberized suits; they lie on undulating rollers and get bounced around by vibrators. The latter two gadgets are supposed to roll or jiggle the fat away. Well, the fat rolls and jiggles, but it doesn't go away.

Another person may do 250 sit-ups each day for two months. His stomach muscles may be tighter but he hasn't lost the fat. The fat remains above the muscles and creates a flabby appearance.

You see, fat does not belong just to your abdomen, hips, buttocks or thighs. Fat belongs to your *entire* body. The only way that fat is going to disappear from a specific region is if the body's caloric demand is so great that the fat is consumed as fuel.

The solution? Aerobic exercise! That form of exercise will tax the largest group of muscles. And through aerobics general body fat, including the problem areas (hips, thighs, etc.), will decrease. The nonaerobic exercises for the particular areas are for stretching and toning up. This combination of exercises will *work.*

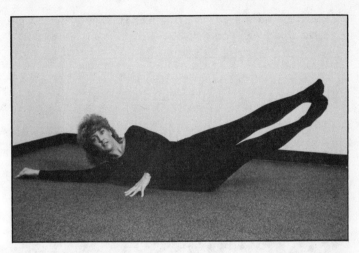

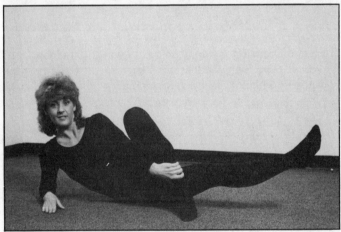

1. Lie on your right side with your right arm outstretched to support you. Raise your left leg in the air. Now bring your right leg up to your left leg. Lower your right leg but leave your left leg up. Now raise the right leg again. Raise, and

lower the right leg 8 to 10 times. Turn over and do the same thing with your left leg.

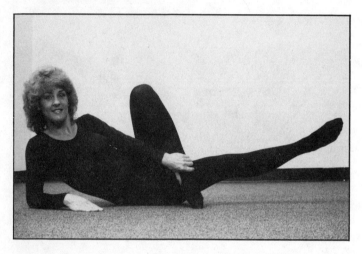

2. Rest on your right side, leaning on your right elbow. Hold your left foot with your left hand and bring it in front of your right leg which is extended an inch above the floor. Now lift your right leg as high as you can. Lower it. Do 10 repetitions. Turn over and do the other leg.

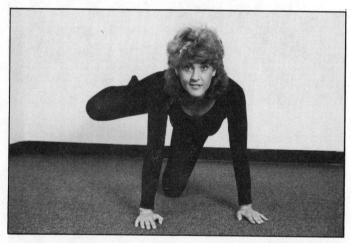

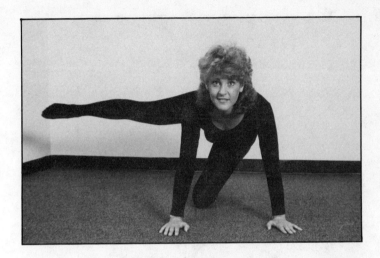

3. Get on your hands and knees with your weight evenly distributed. With back straight, stomach pulled in and your head up, swing your right knee out to the side. From your bent-knee position, swing the rest of your leg out until it is completely straight. Bring leg back to bent-knee position and then lower leg. Try not to move your hips as you lift your knee. Do 10 to 15. Increase until you can do from 35 to 50.

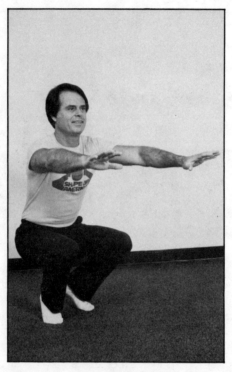

4. The classic "squat" exercise is simple. Stand straight with legs about six inches apart. Bend from the knees and squat down as you extend your arms forward (to aid your balance). Stand again. Breathe deeply and naturally. Repeat this procedure 10 to 15 times until you can do it 50 times. Keep your upper body straight. Don't bend at the waist, only at the knees.

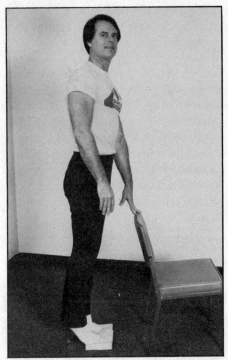

5. Your arches and lower legs will like this exercise. Stand
   behind a straight-back chair with your toes on a book or a
   thick piece of wood. Keep your head up, stomach in and
   your hips forward. Now raise up as high as you can on your
   toes, keeping your heels together. If you haven't done this
   exercise before, your muscles may get sore or cramped but
   the soreness will work out if you regularly do this exercise.
   Do this until it hurts a bit or until you feel "burn."

If you develop sore muscles, soak in a tub of hot water.
This will relieve the soreness. On the next day, make sure you
do some exercises to utilize the same muscles. Do a lot of light
stretching exercises. These will help work out the stiffness. The
soreness will go away in a day or so. There is nothing to worry
about.

To help avoid getting muscle cramps, warm up properly. Also, make sure there is an adequate supply of calcium and potassium in your diet. But, if you get a muscle cramp in your leg, try to stand on it. If it is in other parts of your body, massage and stretch that area for two to three minutes, even if it causes pain. If soreness lasts for quite a while afterward, place warm packs on the area. This will relax the muscle.

If you *pull* a muscle or *sprain* an ankle, *ice it. Don't apply heat* and don't use the area that is injured. Have it checked by a physician. We have a friend who once thought he had only sprained his ankle, so he didn't have it checked. "I'll tough it out," he said with a grimace. Three days later he discovered it was broken. It took twice as long to heal because it wasn't treated immediately.

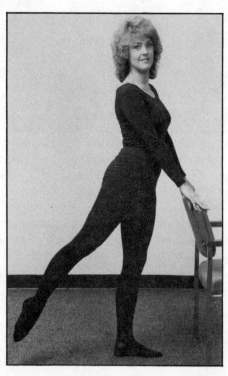

6. This is a leg-extension exercise which will benefit the back part of the hips. Stand behind a chair and place your hands on the back of the chair for proper support. Keep your head up and arch your back. Extend your leg straight back, pointing your toes, first one leg, then the other one. Don't lean forward. Extend each leg 10 times. Relax. Now 10 more times, only a bit faster. Maintain proper posture. Progress to 20 repetitions for each leg.

Chest (Pectorals)

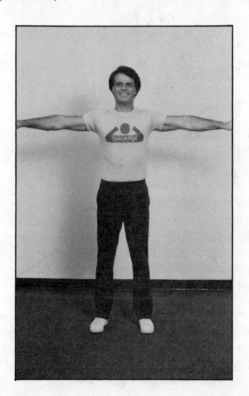

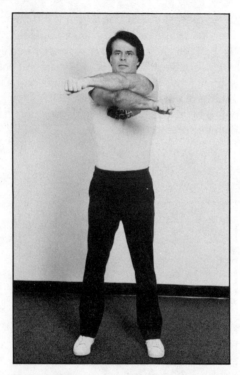

1. Stand with your feet about 12 inches apart and your arms held straight out at your sides. Slowly cross your arms, right over left, pulling each across your chest as far as possible. Return to original position. On the next repetition, cross left over right, and continue to alternate through this set for 10 repetitions. Increase until you can do 20.
2. Lie down on the floor, your hands level with your chest and a little more than shoulder-width apart. Push up with your hands flat, keeping your back straight, and push until your arms are fully extended. Return to original position. Do 8 or 10, and work up to 25 repetitions. Breathe deeply as you do this, in the nose and out of the mouth.

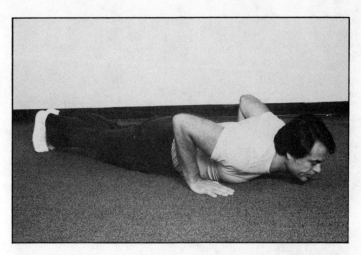

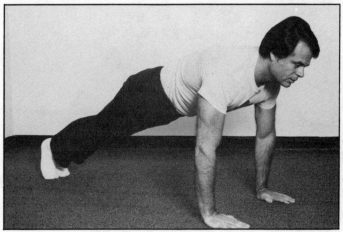

3. The "prone fly" exercise is also good for the chest. Lie on your back. Hold two large (equal weight) books, or very light dumbbells, in each hand. Stretch your arms out perpendicular to your body, then lift them a couple of inches off the

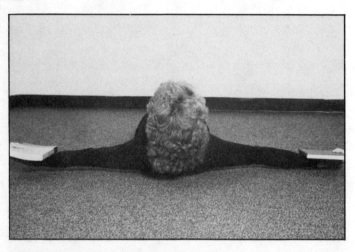

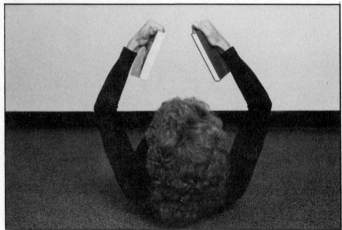

ground. Bring your arms up toward each other, bowing them slightly as if you were hugging a tree. Touch the books together. Keep your chest tense during this exercise. Lower your arms slowly (but don't touch the floor) and relax your chest at the same time. Repeat another 8 or 9 times. Work up to 20 repetitions.

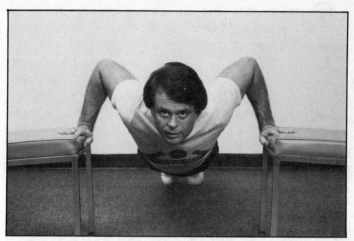

4. This is a variation of the push-up, and a bit harder, for you will be pushing up from two chairs or two benches. Let your body down so that your chest drops *below* your hands,

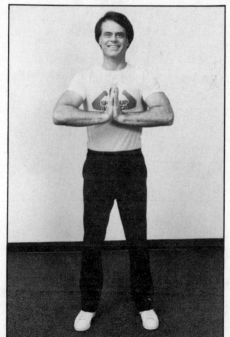

then push back up until your arms are fully extended. Keep your back straight through this exercise. Do 10 or 12 repetitions and work up to 20 repetitions.

5. Stand with your palms together, fingers pointing up, hands about six inches in front of your chest. Press your hands together for 5 to 7 seconds. Relax. Repeat four more times. Lower your arms and relax, shaking your arms. Do three more repetitions. This is an isometric exercise.

Arms

1. Place your feet about six inches apart and hold a book in each hand. Bend your knees and bend forward, keeping your back flat and arms close to your sides. Bring your el-

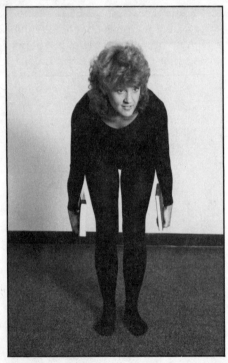

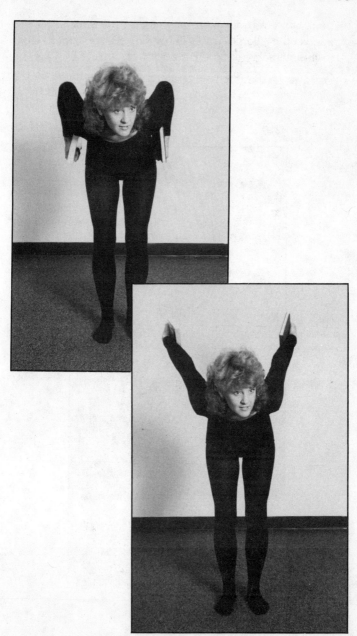

bows up, level with your back, then raise your arms and hands up as high as possible behind your back, then return to the starting position. Do a total of 10 or 12 of these.

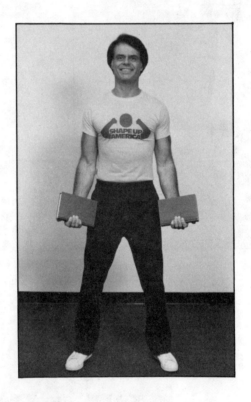

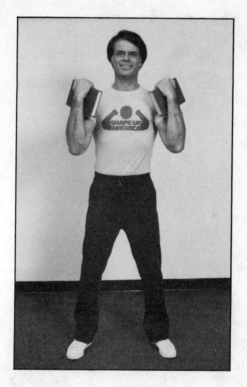

2. Stand straight with your feet about 12 inches apart. Have two evenly-weighted books, or dumbbells, in your hands, down at your sides. Slowly bend your elbows, bring the weights up until they almost touch your shoulders. Lower slowly. Breathe normally, but deeply. Do two sets of 10 each.

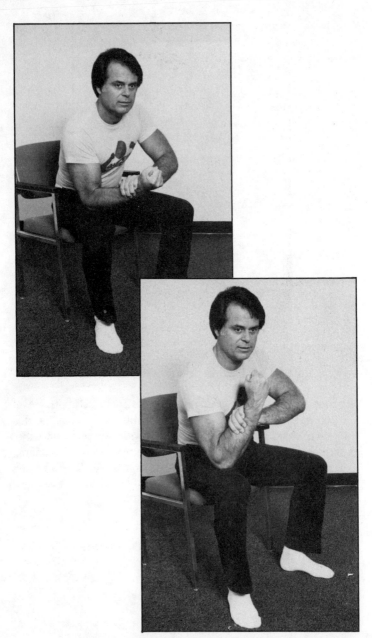

3. This "resistance curl" is known as a bicep-concentration exercise. Sit in a chair with your left elbow on your leg, close to your knee. Take hold of your left wrist with your right hand and "resist" with that hand as your left hand tries to "curl" its way up to the chin. Keep the pressure on that curling arm all the way up so it has to work to get up there. Do 10 repetitions with your left arm. Then switch and work your right arm for 10 repetitions.

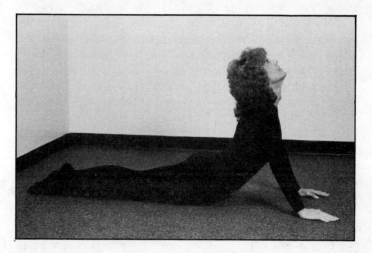

Back

An excellent back exercise is the "cobra stretch." Lie down facing the floor, with your hands by your shoulders, palms down. Now lift your shoulders, helping as little as possible with your hands. Lift until your chest then stomach are off the floor. Look up at the sky and hold that back arch for three seconds. Slowly lower your body. Do this exercise 7 or 8 times and progress to 20 times.

You should do these exercises six days a week either to tone up or stay toned. Prevent boredom by doing them with someone, or by watching TV or listening to recordings. But whatever you do, *do them*! And you'll be on your way to being free to be fit.

Facial Isometrics

Since even before Ponce de Leon searched for the Fountain of Youth, people have been looking for potions, preparations and procedures to remove the signs of aging and restore the appearance they had 20 or 30 years earlier.

Women and men alike are going to plastic surgeons for face lifts and skin abrasions to get rid of bags, lines, valleys and scars. Some are having their skin frozen off by cyrosurgery in order to grow new skin. Some rejuvenation procedures involve having substances placed on the face for days at a time and lying immobile until they are removed. Off comes old skin. This is called "skin peeling."

Has nature relinquished the ability to retain a youthful look to plastic surgeons? Of course not. And when *we* exercise this ability, it is far less painful than the surgeon's way and far more beneficial. People who go the surgery route endure days, weeks and even months of discomfort and incapacitation. They spend thousands of dollars for benefits that are often short-lived.

On the other hand, slowing down the effects of aging *naturally* involves no discomfort, no loss of time, no monetary expense, no phony ego highs and no guilt trips. With little effort, your facial muscles can be brought back to life!

Our facial muscles, as all our muscles, are geared to movement. Natural movements of those muscles assist circulation. Different facial positions revive these functions when facial isometrics are utilized. A "de-activated" face is a deteriorating face. But an "activated" face is being rejuvenated.

When bags form under the eyes and remain, when extra folds of skin collects under the chin, when vertical lines form on the upper lip—these are signs of aging. Aging means deterioration. In these cases, deterioration is of the small muscles that hold the flesh firm, and of the skin that loses its elasticity.

Would you like to do your face a favor right now, without even putting the book down? Would you like to delay the deterioration of your facial muscles and restore some of their efficiency, if deterioration has already begun? We will now do several facial isometric exercises. We will simply use facial "expressions" in a highly constructive manner.

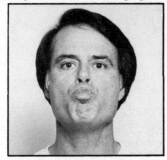 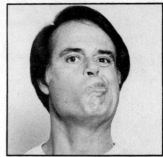

1. Purse your lips as if inviting a kiss. Slowly move them to the left, then back to the starting point. Now move them to the right, then back to the starting point. Rest, then repeat. Do this several times. Make sure you are not moving your lower jaw. Let the tiny muscles around the lips do the work; it keeps them young and elastic.

   Some voluntary muscles actually atrophy through disuse. You will prevent this atrophy around the mouth by doing this exercise daily.

2. Tighten the muscles on each side of your nose as if you felt a yawn or a sneeze coming on. Increase this tension as much as you can. Now let go. Repeat a few times

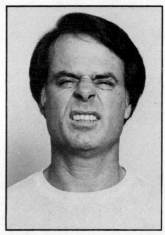

daily. Notice how easy it is and how good it feels.

This exercise restores suppleness to the cheek muscles that border the nose. It helps delay or erase those sag lines that curve around the mouth from the area above the nostrils, sometimes all the way to the chin.

3. Open your eyes as wide as you can and stare. Now look to the left and hold as you count to five. Now look to the right and count to five. Look up and hold. Look down and hold. The tiny muscles around the eyes need your help to remain supple. This exercise keeps the eyelids and area around the eyes elastic.

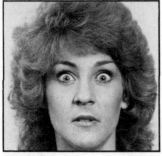 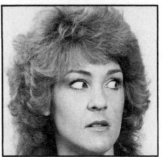

4. Open your mouth as wide as you can. Now hold. Check in a few seconds to see if you can open it still wider. Good. Hold for a few more seconds. Now close. Relax.
5. Pull down your lower lip by tightening the necessary muscle. In effect you are "showing your teeth," but the lower ones only. Feel the neck muscle tense. Now let go. Repeat seven times.

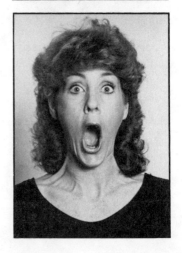

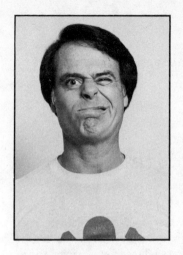 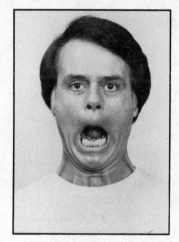

6. Pull the right corner of your mouth up as if in a sneer. Hold. Let go. Now do the same with the left corner. Repeat seven times.

These six simple isometric exercises are "face toners." They make you look younger because they restore vitality to the muscles and tissues you involve. If you find it difficult to control one or two of the muscles, such as raising a corner of your mouth into a sneer, you probably need that exercise all the more.

To gain control, try using a mirror. It acts as a "biofeedback device." You can see results when you do something right. You can even learn to move your ears, your scalp and other "immovables"! Besides, it's a lot of fun to watch yourself make ridiculous faces in the glass.

When you move your muscles, your organs and your tissues, you wake them up. They respond with added life, energy and well-being. By adding life to your years, you are adding years to your life! And more years mean a longer, more productive life of Kingdom service.

"Do you not know that your body is a temple of the Holy Spirit within you, which you have from God? You are not your own; you were bought with a price. So glorify God in your body" (1 Cor. 6:19, 20, RSV).

Chapter Five

BEFORE YOU BEGIN YOUR EXERCISE PROGRAM

The information in this chapter does not anticipate *every* possible situation. But though quite general in nature, we strongly recommend that you carefully read each point and apply it to your situation.

1. Get Medical Approval

If you are over 35 years old, we suggest that you have a complete physical examination before beginning a program. If you are under 35 and have a history of cardiovascular disease, diabetes, hypertension or kidney disease, make sure you consult your doctor. Let your doctor know that you are about to begin a program; and indicate what sort of a program it is— running, weight lifting, bicycle riding, tennis, etc.

If you fit either of these categories, and are going to start a vigorous exercise program such as one of the aerobics, we recommend that you have a *stress electrocardiogram* (EKG). This is different from a routine EKG. Often an EKG will be a *resting* EKG. A stress EKG is performed on a motorized treadmill. Instruments control the amount of exercise and monitor your body while you exercise. If you have any problem within your cardiovascular system, the tests should indicate how serious the problems are and your physician can make recommendations about what type of exercise would be best for you.

2. Fitness Is for a Lifetime

Look upon exercise as a lifetime matter. Fitness is not a goal only for professional athletes. Nor should the goal simply be a quick shape-up. This will be emphasized later in the nutrition section. Fitness is defined by the President's Council on Physical Fitness as "the ability to carry out daily tasks efficiently with enough energy left over to enjoy leisure time pursuits and to meet unforeseen emergencies." The better shape we are in, the more efficiently we function in all areas of our lives.

3. Begin Gradually

A friend of ours decided one day that he was going to get back into shape. He bought running shoes, new socks, put on his old college track outfit and headed for the local high school track. Thinking of his college days, he decided to put in a quick mile as a warm-up.

He made it through one lap, grabbed the nearest bench, collapsed, and promptly threw up. He was angry and embarrassed. He headed home, saying, "Nuts to this. I don't need this at all!"

Fortunately our friend reconsidered. After a slow start the next time out, he got hooked on jogging. Today he runs three miles every morning and regularly plays racquetball with his wife. But it took him four months to get to the point where he could do that much on a regular basis.

Do not overwork yourself when you begin to exercise. Build up *gradually*. Work at your own speed and capacity. Don't try to keep up with someone who has been exercising longer. But don't compromise, either, and fall into the "just get by" syndrome. Remember, the sauna, steam room and whirlpool at the health club are part of the relaxation *after* exercise; they are not in themselves a form of exercise!

4. Enjoy Yourself

Remember that exercise should be challenging *and fun*. Choose activities that you enjoy. If you don't like to run, after a few times you will quit. This happens to approximately 90% of all those who start. No matter how good it may be for you, if you don't *like* to run, it will be very difficult to stick with it. So try something else instead.

You may also need to have some variety in your program. Otherwise you will become bored. So occasionally do things differently. Instead of running the same old route, search out a new one—as you run. Instead of your usual walk, try roving some day, and see how far you can go. Dr. Thomas Bassler, the pathologist whom we mentioned earlier, takes off weekly on a 25-mile walk. He stops for lunch or a snack along the way, frequently breaks into a jog, and the rest of the time just ambles along at an enjoyable pace. He insists that just to walk that far in *any* length of time pushes the heart, lungs and leg muscles to a good, healthy limit.

5. Exercise Regularly

A weekend tennis match or a Saturday afternoon walk will not get you in shape. Fitness is maintained *only* if you exercise at least *three days a week*. Fitness is remarkably improved if you exercise six days a week. Aim for at least 12 minutes a day of an aerobic exercise, and supplement this with other forms of exercise.

Often, weekend sports buffs hurt themselves by pulling muscles or by getting stiff and sore. Demands put on an out-of-shape body often result in pain. If you are just beginning, three days a week, every other day is fine. But as your fitness improves, build up to six days a week. We follow an exercise program for six days, but on the seventh day we do not follow our regular routine. On that seventh day—for us it's Sunday—we do *something different*, in addition to participation in our church activities. Usually this means a bike ride or a walk.

6. Make Exercising Fit Your Schedule

The President's Council on Physical Fitness says everyone needs to exercise at least 30 minutes a day. Just 30 minutes out of 1,440 minutes of a 24-hour day isn't really very much. Some people only have that much time in their schedules. If you don't, then you are just *too* busy. If you have more time, plan a variety of exercises and scatter them throughout your day.

You must adjust your exercise program according to your schedule. Figure out your 24-hour cycle and work exercise into your personal routine. The importrant thing is to set a time to exercise *every* day. Use the DDD method which General Douglas MacArthur announced during World War II: "*Dedication Demands Discipline.*" If you are dedicated to having your bodily Temple become clean and active and full of vitality, then that dedication demands you be disciplined to it. Let *nothing* stop you!

Consider exercising the first thing in the morning before your day's work or school schedule begins. If you do choose morning, remember you will need a longer warm-up period. You need to gradually increase your pulse rate and stretch your muscle groups.

Noontime is good for city workers who have exercise facilities nearby. It breaks up the day and leaves the evenings free. Often a game of volleyball or basketball at the YMCA, or racquetball or squash at the racquet court, or weight lifting or swimming at the spa, will get a person through the afternoon without having that "draggy" feeling.

Many people like to work out in the early evenings because it helps relieve the day's tensions. Instead of feeling so tired, they become alert and invigorated for the evening. They go to bed refreshed and sleep more soundly. Some enjoy a workout right after returning home from work. They say it helps reduce stresses of the day, revives them and also aids them in weight reduction—they aren't as hungry for dinner.

7. Warm Up Properly

Spend from five to seven minutes warming up. If your feel really stiff, you should take a little longer. You also need to spend the same amount of time after you are *finished* with your activity. You need to stretch the muscles out after a workout so they don't remain shortened. If you don't stretch them, you can easily pull a muscle. After running, slow your pace to a jog, then a fast walk, then a regular walk. Don't come to a screeching halt with smoke pouring from your running shoes. If you stop abruptly, the blood collects in your extremities. This is called "pooling." This deprives the heart and brain of needed blood and oxygen, and you may end up with dizziness and even fainting. When you slow down gradually, your muscles help pump the blood back from the extremities to the heart.

8. Record Your Progress

You may want to keep a record of your exercise activities. Record books for runners are available at most bookstores and you can easily convert one to a daily record of other activities which make up your exercise program. You can even use a diary for this.

A daily record keeps you aware of what you have done over the weeks, months, and even years. If you want to set goals for yourself, this is a great way to keep track of progress made toward them.

As part of your daily exercise record, you may want to keep other bits of information about your life. Write down how you feel. Write down what happened during the day. Write down what you hope will happen soon. Write down what the Lord is telling you daily as you spend time with Him.

At the end of the year you can look back on your diary of

your physical and spiritual growth and see that you have become a more disciplined, committed and fit person.

Vince Lombardi, the legendary coach of the Green Bay Packers football team, abhorred laziness wherever he found it—especially on the playing field. He considered laziness to be a form of cheating. One day he caught Leroy Caffey loafing on a play during a practice session.

"Caffey," he yelled, "if you cheat in practice, you will cheat in a game. And if you cheat in a game, you will cheat for the rest of your life. And *I will not have it!*"

Lombardi knew that failure to live up to your potential is sin. To slide toward mediocrity, ease, or comfort is to accept less for yourself than you ought to accept.

There are many tempting things that will present themselves to you as substitutes for the time you might normally spend exercising. It is important that you not be diverted from your program.

"And let us not be weary in well doing: for in due season we shall reap, if we faint not" (Gal. 6:9, KJV).

Chapter Six

RECIPE FOR TOTAL HEALTH

Have you ever stopped to consider some of the feats of physical stamina recorded in the Bible? Joseph walked 50 miles to see his brothers when he was but a teenager (Gen. 37:13-17). The famous Jericho march on the seventh day was a six-mile hike for the people of Israel (Josh. 6:3, 4). Moses, at the age of 120, climbed Pisgah Peak on Mount Nebo (Deut. 34:1). Jesus walked the 50 miles from Gennesaret to Tyre and Sidon (Matt. 15:21). And two of the disciples walked the seven miles from Jerusalem to Emmaus for supper and then hustled back to Jerusalem that same night (Luke 24:13-34).

We easily overlook these rather casual references to physical stamina because we don't consider the distances involved as we read these accounts. But men of biblical times did these things without the aid of the conveniences we have, and they did them as part of ordinary daily living.

These people did not spend time working out, jogging, lifting weights or joining health clubs. How, then, can we account for these instances of robust good health and physical stamina enjoyed by *ordinary* people? Surely one reason is that the people of ancient times never acquired a dependence upon the energy-saving conveniences we have available to us. Therefore, they thought nothing of walking 50 miles or more.

Yet there is surely something more. A significant change has taken place in the last century—a change in thinking, which has resulted in the growth of an artificial world around us. We have become so dependent on this artificiality that we can no longer tolerate the natural conditions which previous generations thrived on. God gave mankind fresh air and the lungs to breathe it. He gave sunlight which gives light, warmth and life. He gave living, natural sources of food. He gave mankind dominion over the fields, streams and woods.

But we humans have attempted to improve upon the world that God created. We have attempted to improve upon God's laws of physical movement. So instead of walking, we now ride in cars, trains or airplanes. Instead of picking something up and carrying it, we build a machine to do it for us at the press of a switch. And instead of eating food which God has made to grow naturally, we refine, dilute, process, package, color, refrigerate, freeze, dry and then reprocess. And we do it all in the name of civilization, convenience and progress. Today civilization is measured by how much ease accompanies living. Those who can sit the most and enjoy artificial rather than natural things are considered the most advanced. We live in a society that has been seduced by artificial foods, artificial air, artificial light and artificial entertainment.

No wonder we are run-down, tuckered out, and always ready for another vacation! Americans annually spend $217.9 billion on health care alone—almost 10% of the gross national product. Physicians pocketed $46.6 billion of that total. We spend $19.2 billion on drugs to help us get up in the morning, hold out through the day, and relax enough in the evening so that we can get some sleep. Then the next day we repeat the cycle.

We would like to reverse the downward spiral. We would like to help you to return to total good health by returning, not only to physical exercise, but to natural nutrition as well.

We believe that nature provides the recipe for total health. This recipe is no recent development. It dates from the creation of the world. And it is not a result of human genius. *God* reveals in His creation the life-style which leads to total health. We can ignore it, distort it, alter it and debase it. Or we can follow it. The recipe provides for the wellness of the spirit, mind and body. But because the *body* has been subject to such abuse in our time, we would like to concentrate upon how the body can be restored to health.

God's Laws of Nutrition

Most of us lack even basic knowledge about nutrition. Even physicians learn little about nutrition during medical school studies. One consequence of this general ignorance is that the food production and distribution in the United States is largely exempt from nutritional controls. Nearly anything can be sold as food. All one has to do is convince people to eat it. And a huge advertising industry makes millions of dollars doing just that. In fact, nearly all food production is governed by *commercial* considerations, which have to do with what will stay on shelves without spoiling, and what will turn the most profit for processors, handlers and retailers. Nutrition seems to be the last consideration of most people who produce most of the food we normally eat.

God established laws which regulate His creation. He designed the world to work according to His precise plan. But when we ignore God's natural laws of health, we gradually destroy our bodies. Man has woven into God's world many artificial, unnatural things. Mankind's doings are imprecise and imperfect. Therefore, human efforts often interfere with God's perfect design.

What are some violations of God's natural laws? How do the artificial products of mankind violate the natural laws of God? Well, let's take a look at food common to nearly every American kitchen. There are sugary cereals; baked goods made from refined flour; packaged and pre-cooked foods containing chemical preservatives, dyes and other additives; and soft drinks containing artificial sweeteners and caffeine. And the list can go on and on. But all are human creations. All are artificial. All are attempts by humans to improve upon God's creation.

God did not give us white refined flour. He gave us *whole grain* which is "alive," which contains the bran and germ.

God did not give us white sugar. He gave us sugar cane, from which flows a natural, nutritious, sweet syrup.

God did not give us french-fried potatoes. He gave us the natural potato that can be baked or steamed without added fat.

We believe that when God calls us to be His children, He calls us to return to a life lived according to His pattern. And in the pages that follow we would like to spell out for you what this pattern might indicate concerning proper nutrition. It may require some stubborn effort on your part to change your eating and cooking habits. And you may have to endure some ridicule to do it—even a slight deviation from the status quo may cause others to label you as a "health-food fanatic." But which is most important, doing things God's way or trying to please others? We believe the blessings of doing things God's way far outweigh the "benefits" of people-pleasing.

"And so, dear brothers, I plead with you to give your bodies to God. Let them be a living sacrifice, holy—the kind He can accept. When you think of what He has done for you, is this too much to ask? Don't copy the behavior and customs of this world, but be a new and different person with a fresh newness in all you do and think. Then you will learn from your own experience how His ways will really satisfy you" (Rom. 12:1, 2, TLB).

Chapter Seven

FITNESS AND WEIGHT CONTROL

We've perpetuated an age-old myth which says that fat people are jolly people. But is it "jolly" to always sit uncomfortably? To always breathe heavily, huffing and puffing after climbing a short flight of stairs? To have to be tugging continually at one's clothing as it cuts into one's waistline? To feel self-conscious about one's appearance whenever other people are around? Can you live a long and healthy life carrying 20, 50, or more pounds of excess weight?

Statistics show that overweight people suffer more disease and risk dying sooner than people of normal weight. According to the Metropolitan Life Insurance Company, a person 10 pounds overweight at the age of 45 or older decreases his chance of survival by 8%. With each additional pound, his/her risk of dying prematurely rises 1%. Many health insurance companies charge overweight people higher premiums due to their increased chances of physical problems.

The first commandment states, "Thou shalt have no other gods before me." Many Christians walking around with bulging bellies announce to the world that they do, indeed, have another god in their life—*food*. And even the best of food is pollution for the body if taken in excess, or if it is used as a psychological or spiritual crutch.

Food sometimes serves the same purpose as tobacco, alcohol or drugs. When feeling anxious, some people automatically reach for something to eat. When confronting a challenge, they immediately search for food. When responding to depression or disappointment, they immediately start eating. And excessive eating shows its pollution on the *outside* of the body. It makes people fat.

Satan and the Stout

"Get thee behind me, Satan," a person frequently says, when tempted to eat sugary, fattening, or simply too much food. Too often Satan obeys—and gives them a push from behind!

Satan wants Christians out of control. And food is an easy device for him to use to get them out of control. Most Christians do not think of food as something which pollutes, damages and kills. After all, a person has to eat. So what could be sinful about food? So the devil merely has to get us to eat more—more of something we like. We then end up living to eat rather than eating to live. We therefore eat more snacks and larger meals. Soon gluttony is upon us without our even being aware that we are committing sin.

Webster's dictionary defines gluttony as "the habit of eating too much." It isn't necessary to weigh 300 pounds to do that. We have a friend who appears to be normal weight. Yet at almost every meal he overeats. He literally stuffs himself with food, then moves uncomfortably to the front-room couch and lies down to get some relief. Most people think that, since he doesn't *appear* to be overweight, he must be just a "hearty eater." Those same people would frown if they saw an obviously overweight person eating the same amount of food. But gluttony is gluttony, regardless of the eater's size. Consider these strong words written by Paul: ". . . many live as *enemies of the cross of Christ.* Their destiny is destruction, *their God is their stomach,* and their glory is in their shame" (Phil. 3:18, 19, NIV).

Frankly, Satan does not care if we are fat or thin. He cares only that we are under the control of our appetites, which includes our appetite for food. But fatness almost always follows gluttony: "Be sure your sin will find you out." And with fatness we are changed not only physically, but mentally, emotionally and even spiritually. We lack vigor. We tend to procrastinate. We think of food when we should be thinking of prayer and worship. We even lose our self-respect, because we know that we are out of control. And soon we lose the respect of others.

When Satan gains a foothold on our will, we become bound by food. God doesn't want us to be bound by anything and that includes food. God knows that when an area of our physical desires is out of control, it can actually compete with our love for God (Phil. 3:19).

But we can regain control over our appetites through the power of the Holy Spirit. God wants us to become disciplined, to master all of our appetites. Discipline is necessary to our Christian walk. And when we think of the serious consequences of excess weight, we see it is also necessary for our survival.

But we are going to need God's help to regain control and to lose weight. He will not melt those ugly pounds away magically. Neither will He remove the desire for food—we need food to survive. But He will help us to help ourselves, not to a second portion, but to *moderation.* He wants us to master our appetite so *we* have control over it rather than it having control over us.

Before you read on, put this book down and pray. Tell God you want to regain control of your appetite, and to restore your body to natural health. Yield all of your appetites to Him. You may want to claim John 14:13, 14, and make those foundational verses as you depend on the Lord's strength to gain this victory.

The High Cost of Excess Weight

Overeating, eating the wrong foods, and inactivity comprise the "big three" reasons for obesity in America. It may be one of them or all three that trouble you. Obesity has been shown to contribute to a number of serious health problems, including:

high blood pressure
coronary heart disease
gall bladder disorders
diabetes
joint and bone problems
kidney trouble
chronic indigestion

But the problems aren't just physical ones. Consider the high costs incurred by obesity.

The Cost of Obesity in the U.S.
(1976 figures)

Doctor's fees	$238 million
Hospital costs	32 million
Medications	157 million
Weight-reduction clubs	61 million
Total costs for obesity	$488 million

These outrageous costs continue to mount each year. But an overweight person's costs usually end quickly—more quickly than he expects: death strikes prematurely.

Often the fat person dies prematurely because many medical procedures hold increased risks for a fat person. A normally routine medical procedure on an obese person often becomes complicted and risky. Surgery, for instance, on an overweight person can be accompanied by more postoperative complications. An overweight person is also more prone to accidents because of his lessened agility and slower reflexes. A fat woman who wants to have children may find that her obesity is a factor in her infertility. And if a fat woman becomes pregnant, the statistical probability of birth complications rises significantly.

When a person is overweight he has too much body fat. But you do not have to be overweight to have excess fat on your body. A simple test to check this is to pinch yourself *under* your upper arm—not your bicep, but your tricep area. If your fingers are able to grip more than one inch of flesh, the excess is fat.

Another way to test this is to see how easily you can float in a swimming pool. The more easily you float, the more fat you have on your body. We mentioned this at one of our nationally-conducted "Shape Up, America" seminars; a man came up to us during a break and told us that when he was in his 20's he was a trained athlete—lean. He said he used to try to float in a pool and would sink so fast that he would almost hit the bottom and bounce up. Now, 20 years older and 40 pounds heavier, he has no problem floating.

Excess fat can be laced within the muscles (intramuscular fat). "Overweight" fat lies between the muscle and the skin (subcutaneous fat). The latter is the more obvious fat we see, such as the "roll around the middle." But either way, there is too much fat.

When you go on a reducing diet remember that weight loss and fat loss are not necessarily the same. The body cells contain water and other nutrients, along with fat. In the first couple of days much of the weight loss will be water loss and not fat loss. That is why some people tend to drop the initial weight so quickly. But losing a pound of water weight is not really a true weight loss as it will be regained almost as quickly as it came off. What you really want is fat loss. Often that loss will show up in loss of inches rather than in loss of pounds. If you replace intramuscular fat with muscle, you won't lose any weight, but you'll lose obvious inches!

Dozens of fad diets have been published in the past 20 years. If you believe them all, you would eat mostly protein; or you would eat mostly fat; or you would eat mostly carbohydrates; or you would brush your teeth instead of eating; or you would eat only brown rice; or you would eat only grapefruit and carrot sticks; or you would eat only one meal a day; or you would eat six meals a day.

All of the diets work. Fad diets work because they restrict the calorie intake and lower the water content in the tissue. There may also be some muscle loss. But you cannot stay on those diets safely for any length of time because they are nutritionally unbalanced *and* they are harmful to your body.

The fad diets will have you lose weight, all right, but *keeping* the weight off is another ballgame. Here is where most of the diet plans seem to fail. As we mentioned, a lot of the loss was water and muscle, and not fat. Quite often, too, when someone is on one of these extreme diets, all that person is thinking about is getting off the diet. The diet is looked upon as a time of deprivation and when the diet is over he will unhesitatingly return to his destructive eating pattern: diet, lose weight, revert to old eating habits, regain weight, diet, etc. The cycle never seems to cease.

Mary, age 32, told us she had lost 425 pounds in a five-year period! She had dieted ten times, and each time she lost over 40 pounds. But she gained it back each time, and usually gained more than she had lost. She finally decided to stop all the fad diets and began to eat the natural food plan which we will give you in the next chapter. She also embarked on an exercise program similar to the one we proposed earlier. She began to lose weight/fat in a healthy manner, and kept it off. She is in terrific shape today and praising the Lord for it.

Repeated weight gains and losses shock your body. Yet millions of people do this to themselves every year. We call it the "yo-yo syndrome"—up and down, up and down. We'd like to include a brief warning about the serious consequences of such extremes as self-induced vomiting and rigid dieting for prolonged periods (teenage girls are extremely susceptible to such practices).

"As many as 30 percent of all college women suffer from two diet-associated diseases—*anorexia nervosa* and *bulimarexia,*" says Washington State University psychologist, Barbara Merriam. Starvation is the main characteristic of anorexia nervosa, and it seems to begin most often in adolescent years. It mainly afflicts girls (who may be rejecting womanhood). Less than 5% of anorexics are males. The person with this disease dangerously restricts her calorie intake, and in some cases, stops eating completely. Usually this person will overexercise so she can burn off calories rapidly. This practice can be fatal if not stopped.

Bulimarexia ("binge eating") is when the person eats massive quantities of food in a short period of time. The person then purges herself through vomiting or laxatives. The food she consumes will be very high in calories—often "junk food," and she prefers to eat alone. She will also stay off food by fasting for a couple of days, so there is frequent weight fluctuation. This disorder tends to begin in the late teens.

We know a woman who has suffered from this. She has actually consumed about 6,000 calories in one sitting: three hamburgers, two milk shakes, two containers of french fries, one quart of ice cream, an entire chocolate cake, three candy bars and a whole pie. She would eat until she was so stuffed she literally couldn't move.

Both the bulimarexic and the anorexic have an exaggerated fear of getting fat. Their practices often begin after a successful diet as means of keeping the weight off. The bulimarexics tend to be perfectionists and extroverts. Most of them have been heavy at one time. The anorexics are usually more introvertive and shy. Bulimarexics appear to be healthy, vigorous and maintaining normal weight, but anorexics look like skeletons.

Both types have a distorted body image. Both need treatment, medically and psychologically. The key is probably a matter of spiritual bondage. If you are suffering from either of these disorders or know someone who is, please see a doctor and a counselor. There *is* help!

Getting Started

You're thinking, "Well, yeah, maybe I should do something about it, but..."

No more excuses! There have been too many already.

To begin losing weight, you must admit you *are* over-weight and that you want to do something about it. Cast aside the memories of all those other times you tried to lose weight and failed. That is past history. Today is *now*. Because of past failures you may hate yourself and think of yourself as a "fat failure." But you need to look upon yourself as God does. He does not hate you and He does not consider you a failure. You can accept yourself just as God does—unconditionally. God *wants* you to lose weight. He knows how unhealthy this condition is for you. He will help you win this battle. But you've got to *want* it!

Say to yourself, "*This* time I will succeed with God's help—by His grace through my works!"

Permanent weight loss can be yours without an enslaving, restrictive diet plan; without special charts to memorize; without scales to stand on (and lie about); without the danger of gaining all the weight back as soon as you get off a diet.

What we are presenting, in this chapter and the next, is *not* a diet. It is a plan, a way of life, that you can use *the rest of your life.* You will be consuming natural foods that taste good. They are the foods that God gave us to enjoy.

Food itself is not the enemy. The enemy is the *type* of food you eat, and the *amount* you eat. Realize that food is your "fuel." You want the best fuel possible to power your "machine"—your body. Why should you settle for anything less than the best?

The foods you eat need to contain adequate amounts of protein, vitamins and minerals, carbohydrates and essential fatty acids. Refined foods such as white sugar, white flour, hydrogenated fats do not contain the ingredients you need for good health. These are foods that will put fat on the body and can easily make up 60% of your calorie intake. Do you realize what will happen if you remove them and replace them with natural foods, such as whole grains, lean poultry and fish, fresh fruits and vegetables? *You will lose weight!*

The only way you can lose weight, keep it off and have

better health is by decreasing your calorie intake, by being concerned about the type (quality) of food you are eating and by increasing your exercise. It's so simple—and it works!

We are not going to make you a slave to a calorie chart. Too often we find people, who are trying to lose weight, bound to their calorie charts. They are mistakenly focusing on the calories and ignoring the quality of the food. Some of the chart watchers will eat one almond and then sprint to the chart to see how many calories they have swallowed. They gasp and never eat another almond for the rest of their lives. Yvonne used to delete whole food groups such as breads and cereals, which are full of fiber, vitamins and minerals, because she thought they were too high in calories. In their place she would indulge in chemical-laden substitute foods, such as low calorie soft drinks. Yvonne was not only damaging her body, she was depriving it of nutrition. Suppose she had been offered a handful of sunflower seeds or a handful of chocolate-chip cookies. She would quickly calculate that the sunflower seeds contained 350 calories and the cookies held only 275. Therefore, she would eat the cookies, a tragic mistake. The sunflower seeds would have furnished her more food value for the calories and the food would have been utilized by her body. The cookies, however, being full of sugar, would have turned to fat in her body. Body cells are not fooled. They don't count calories; they count nutrients.

Some of you are saying, "But I want some kind of guideline. How many calories can I get *down* to?" Fair enough. If you're a woman, you should not go below 1,200, and if you're a man, you should not go below 1,600. Any daily calorie intake below these figures will guarantee inadequate nutrition. Some of the crazy fad diets put people on a near-starvation diet of 600 to 700 calories. Some go even lower. These diets can defeat your purpose. When you go below 600 calories, your metabolic rate can slow down so much that instead of losing fat, you will lose muscle. That is genuine starvation.

Exercise and Weight Loss

Diet alone will take off some weight. Exercise alone will not result in much weight loss. But combine diet and exercise and you will have a powerful weight-loss team.

The U.S. Department of Health, Education and Welfare states in their book on obesity that a lack of physical activity encourages obesity in two ways: (1) A very small amount of calories consumed are actually used in energy. The excess is stored as fat deposits in the body. (2) The body has an internal mechanism which regulates the appetite and will tell you when you are full. This mechanism does not function properly when there is a low level of physical exertion.

Most thin people receive these internal cues which tell them when they are hungry and when they're full. Yvonne never used to know what that was like. She would eat in response to *external* cues, such as the smell or appearance of food, the time of day, etc., but not because she was actually hungry. She would usually overeat because she couldn't perceive the internal message which warned that she was full. She also used to gobble her food so quickly (something a lot of overweight people do) that she would have consumed a great deal of food before she actually felt "stuffed."

When we talk about exercise and losing weight, we find many people who immediately rationalize their positions with a rather feeble excuse: "I'll gain weight because exercise will make me hungry." However, several independent studies have shown that *exercise will depress the appetite* for a period of time. Most people have stores of fat in their body. When they exercise, the blood sugar level remains stable, because the muscles will be using fat more readily than the sugar, as fuel.

If you're overweight, here are two important "exercises" you should implement immediately:

(1) *The Pushing Movement:* push away from the table before you have eaten too much.

(2) *The Side-to-Side Movement:* move your head from side-to-side when someone asks if you want a second helping.

Those two proven "exercises" need to be utilized daily, but along with the exercises we gave earlier—especially the aerobic exercises. If you haven't started on an aerobics program, you are already one day behind. Remember, aerobics will remove the fat *within* your muscles, as well as the fat *between* your muscles and your skin.

When people are losing weight they sometimes reach a plateau where they don't seem to lose any weight for a period of time. This occurs because the metabolism slows down. But if you exercise right from the beginning, as well as change your eating patterns, often the plateau can be avoided. When you work the muscles throughout your body, your metabolism "wakes up" and burns fat. This occurs not just while you are exercising but for many hours after you have stopped exercising.

As people grow older, their metabolism naturally slows from what it was when they were in their early 20's. After about the age of 35 it decreases noticeably. If you're in this age bracket, make certain that as you start to decrease your intake of food, you also increase activity, in order to boost your metabolism. Unfortunately, the opposite is usually true for many as they grow older. They keep eating the same portions but decrease their activities.

Faithful exercise, along with the proper eating habits, will make the body firm and help to redistribute the weight more attractively.

We have one friend who didn't feel she needed to exercise while she was trying to lose weight. She has lost about 45 pounds, but her skin hangs on her and her body looks like that of an average 70-year-old woman. She is only 35. She is now frantically trying to rectify what she could have avoided by exercising regularly.

As you exercise daily while you're trying to lose weight, you will gain some self-control in the mental, emotional and spiritual areas of your life. A bonus!

Guidelines for Losing Weight

Here is some help for staying with your new way of eating and living. These guidelines are *not* gimmicks. They will shore up your spiritual, mental and physical resolve to lose weight.

1. *Set reasonable weight-loss goals.* A couple of pounds a week is both safe and achievable. Resist impatience. You have gained excess poundage over a period of years, so don't expect "divine surgery" to instantly remove it and don't attempt a crazy crash program to drop 35 pounds in three weeks.

Your problem began because you ate just a *little* more than you needed each day. A few dozen extra calories aren't really that noticeable. But in a year's time those few daily calories that you didn't burn off can easily add up to several additional and unwanted pounds. You didn't gain the weight overnight, so don't expect to lose it overnight.

2. *Don't skip meals,* especially breakfast. When you skip a meal, your blood sugar drops below the normal level and you can suffer from hypoglycemic symptoms, such as irritability, shakiness, shortened attention span and a huge appetite (especially for sweets). People suffering from hypoglycemia will often, by 4:00 in the afternoon, attempt to eat anything they can get their hands on. They usually end up overeating.

3. *Eat balanced, regular meals.* The best plan to follow for eating is to eat a well-balanced breakfast, lunch and light dinner. Most weight gains occur from eating large meals at night; people are usually inactive at night, and don't exercise enough to burn up the calories consumed. A good motto to remember: *"The later the meal, the lighter the meal."*

4. *Eat in only one place in your home.* Living by the rule that there is only one place to eat cuts down on the number of times you will even think about eating.

5. *Keep extra food in the kitchen.* Dish out the food in the kitchen and then bring the plates to the dining room. This makes taking a second helping much more of a conscious effort.

6. *Avoid the "Clean Plate Club" mentality.* Many of us learned as children that if we ate everything on our plate we would get a reward. Sadly, reward usually was a sugary dessert. This problem can carry over into adulthood. We will tend to overeat because we are always trying to clean off our plates. To avoid this problem, *take smaller portions.* If you become comfortably full and still have food on the plate, just wrap the food, place it in the refrigerator and eat it the next day. Please don't tell your children about all the starving children in other countries; don't force them to eat out of guilt. You will be giving them a warped concept of eating.

In regard to children, consider if you are using food as either a reward or punishment for your children's behavior. Do you ever tell them that if they're good at the dentist's office, you will reward them with an ice cream cone? Or, if they do something wrong that they can't have dessert? Or, if they will behave themselves in the grocery cart, you will buy them a candy bar at the check-out counter? Such "food bribery" can carry over into adulthood. Your children may, as adults, use food to deal with their emotions, often to their detriment.

7. *Make healthy foods most accessible.* Keep fresh vegetables and fruits in the front part of the refrigerator so that they will be the first things you see when you open the door looking for a snack. Eat them rather than cookies and cake.

8. *Plan ahead for "trouble" situations.* If you must eat out or attend a party during your weight-loss time, eat before you leave home. This will curb your appetite so that you can get by eating only a few of the healthier, choice items at the party. In such situations, Yvonne also makes sure to wear something with a snug fitting waistband. This prevents her from eating too much. (The last thing one wants to do in public is struggle to release one's waistband.)

9. *Adding more fiber to your diet.* Fiber is a very bulky food, so you will eat less but feel full. Adding fiber to your diet will also help prevent a problem common to many low-calorie diets—constipation. Many of the foods called for in these diets (e.g., meat, cottage cheese, eggs) do not contain fiber.

Here is an extra bonus! A study conducted by the U.S. Department of Agriculture, in cooperation with the University of Maryland, showed that a diet moderately high in fiber caused the body to absorb about 5% fewer calories than when a typical low-fiber diet was consumed. This occurred with a *moderate* intake of fiber. If you follow the high-fiber health plan we will be giving to you, your percentage of unabsorbed calories could be significantly higher.

10. *Don't give up if you lose a skirmish.* If you blow your eating plan by munching on a brownie, don't say, "Oh, well, to God be the glory," and chow down ten more brownies.

11. *Don't assign someone to be your "conscience."* You will end up eating behind his/her back. Won't you feel a bit embarrassed when you're caught in your tool shed at 10:30 at night, eating Twinkies by flashlight behind your lawn mower?

12. *Lower your fat intake.* Don't cut it out, just cut back. Fat's calories are highly concentrated. One ounce of fat contains 225 calories. One ounce of protein or carbohydrates holds about half that amount.

13. *Provide yourself sweet alternatives.* If you want something sweet to munch on, try frozen grapes, cherries or bananas.

14. *Always shop for groceries after you have eaten a meal.* Never shop just before mealtime. Food displays are designed to attract *hungry* people. If you aren't hungry when you shop, you won't fall for the display.

15. *Expect to succeed.* Stop thinking *fat.* Begin to visualize yourself as *lean.* Forget about your past failures in losing weight. Remind yourself that you are using a natural, nutritious way to reach your goal of proper body weight. And accept yourself and love yourself as God accepts and loves you.

You are not on a fad diet. You are on an eating plan that you will live with for the rest of your life. This is not something temporary. You are changing your eating habits permanently. Aim for proper body size and shape, as well as good health. Don't settle for anything else.

Your reason for such drastic change is not for the purpose of fitting into a new swim suit, or of looking good for the upcoming class reunion. It is for the purpose of *obeying God* and becoming like Christ. You have realized that God cannot be glorified in a temple that is overweight, out of shape and fueled by junk food. And that if your temple is transformed into a worthy dwelling, God is pleased. If you choose to live a disciplined, purposeful life, in accordance with the Scriptures, you will be living exactly as God wants you to. And you will become like Jesus.

"For God has not given us a spirit of timidity, but of power and love and discipline" (2 Tim. 1:7, NASB).

Chapter Eight

TOTAL NUTRITION FOR TOTAL FITNESS

We want to help you return to *total* good health. As you begin to restore natural movement and flexibility to your body, you should also provide natural nutrition to feed the awakening cells of your body.

We are tempted to say that this natural nutrition begins in your supermarket or in your kitchen. But it begins elsewhere. It begins in *you!*

You must decide that you want your body to be a living tribute to God's perfection, an energetic instrument for Kingdom work.

Unfortunately, Americans are the most overfed, overweight and yet *undernourished* nation on earth! Dr. Jean Mayer of Harvard University's Department of Nutrition said, "Malnutrition, whether caused by poverty or improper diet, contributes to the alarming health situation in the United States today."

How can improper diet be rampant in a country that has such an abundance of food? It is because so many people today believe they are eating properly, if they are eating from the "basic four food groups" (milk; fruits and vegetables; meat; breads and cereals). But the food they are eating within those groups may not contain the basics of what is needed for good health.

Proper nutrition is gained from a diet that provides us with all the essential nutrients: protein, carbohydrates, fats, fiber, vitamins, minerals, enzymes and water. Each has a very important function and needs to be supplied daily in adequate amounts.

Eat an apple. You will receive carbohydrates; vitamins A and B; calcium; some phosphorous; iron and a small amount of protein. An apple contains a number of the essential nutrients needed to support good health.

Now eat a spoonful of sugar. It contains nothing but carbohydrates, empty calories. It doesn't nourish your body at all. In fact, it has been shown to harm your body.

If your body is deficient in one nutrient, then your body's delicate clockwork mechanism is thrown out of balance. This can occur when you eat a diet heavy in sugar, white flour, processed and refined foods. This can lead to a multiplicity of problems, from lack of energy to skin problems to degenerative diseases (e.g., arthritis, diabetes, heart disease and cancer).

The maxim "You are what you eat" is often preached by many people in the field of health. It is a true statement. The food you consume directly affects your bodily growth, development and ability to live an energetic life. It affects the quality of your life, in regard to how you work, play, think and feel. When your diet is made up of the foods God gave to us, i.e., fruits, vegetables, whole grains, raw milk, legumes, etc., you experience part of the "abundant life" which God desires us to have. This chapter will teach you which foods to choose as you change to a diet of healthy food.

Protein

Protein's major role is in building and repairing the body. It is also involved with hormone production and with enzymes that control the chemical reactions in the body. Protein is not stored in the body, so you must replenish your body's supply daily.

Proteins are composed of amino acids—22 of them. Fourteen of them are manufactured by the body. The other eight (called essential amino acids) must be derived from the food we eat.

Proteins from animal sources, such as fish, eggs, meat and

dairy products, contain the eight essential amino acids. Vegetable proteins, such as those from beans, grains, seeds and nuts, do not each contain all of the eight essential amino acids. But when the vegetable proteins are properly combined, they will furnish all eight (e.g., combining corn and beans, as used often in Mexican cooking; combining peanut butter and whole wheat bread).

We recommend that you use more vegetable proteins. They're less expensive, and add much variety to your meal planning—there are only about 5 basic kinds of meat, plus poultry, but there are over 24 different types of beans, lentils and grains.

Carbohydrates

Carbohydrates are your body's primary source of energy.

Carbohydrates are divided into two groups: simple and complex. The simple carbohydrates, such as fruits, honey and molasses, can be broken down into sugar/glucose more quickly than the complex carbohydrates. The complex carbohydrates are found in whole grains, vegetables, seeds and beans. Because they break down into glucose more slowly, they can provide you with sustained energy over longer periods of time than the simple carbohydrates can.

We recommend a diet that contains a great deal of complex carbohydrates and a moderate level of simple carbohydrates.

The carbohydrates you'll want to shun are the ones found in refined sugar, refined grains (e.g., white rice), white flour and products containing these. They play havoc with the body and can cause a rapid rise in the delicate blood sugar level. When that happens the pancreas secretes more insulin to remove the excess sugar in the system. Often too much is removed. This will leave you very tired, and possibly with a craving for sweets.

If you are reducing, don't cut way back on your carbohydrate intake. You'll need carbohydrates to properly break down fat stores in your body. These carbohydrates also contain valuable nutrients needed by the body. The only carbohydrates you should cut out are the refined ones. Those are the "bad guys" that put weight on. Refined carbohydrates do not contain fiber, either.

Cellulose, or fiber, is a major carbohydrate group. Fiber is found in the cell walls of whole grains, fruits, vegetables, beans, seeds and nuts. It is the part of the food that is indigestable. After it enters your body, it swells once it has come in contact with liquid. It aids in moving material along quickly through your digestive tract. Most Americans find that their food moves along very slowly and that their systems become quite sluggish. This is a very unhealthy condition. The reason the food moves slowly is that average Americans' diets are highly refined. Thus, they do not receive the proper amount of fiber needed for good health. Unexplainably, most Americans are increasingly avoiding the fiber rich foods.

When there is inadequate fiber in the diet, a person may be a prime candidate for cancer of the colon and rectum, diverticular disease, colitis, constipation, appendicitis, hiatal hernia, hemorrhoids, obesity and diabetes.

Because fiber takes longer to chew, it is an excellent food for dieters. And, as mentioned earlier, it is very filling so the eater can fill up on less food.

How can you include more fiber in your diet? Follow the diet plan we have listed in the following pages and you will be getting plenty of fiber. We will emphasize (1) using whole grains and whole grain products; (2) consuming more fresh fruits and vegetables in their raw, uncooked state (overcooking can break down the fiber), and leaving as many of the skins on these foods as possible; (3) eating beans, seeds and nuts.

Bran, an excellent fiber food, is easy to add to your diet. It is sold as unprocessed or miller's bran. Start out with about two teaspoons a day and increase slowly to about two tablespoons. Mix it into cereal, casseroles, meatloaf, and bread or baked goods. If you are trying to lose weight, we recommend that, along with the plan we will be giving you, you stir one or two teaspoons of bran into water or juice and drink it before each meal. You will find that you won't require as much food.

If you are going to include bran in your diet, here are two points to remember. Make sure you are getting plenty of liquid along with the bran. Also make sure your diet has an adequate supply of calcium; bran is high in phosphorus, and too much can actually deplete your body's supply of calcium.

Fats

Fats are your body's second most important source of energy. Fats also carry the fat-soluble vitamins, A, D, E and K, throughout the body. Fats will help keep your skin healthy, and provide essential fatty acids.

Fats are a highly concentrated food. They contain nine calories per gram—twice as much as protein or carbohydrates contain per gram. Carefully limit your intake of fats, especially if you are trying to lose weight.

The average American's diet has shifted from a diet low in fat to one that is high. He consumes between 40% and 45% of his daily calorie intake as fats. This should be lowered to 15% to 20%. Acquaint yourself with the types of fats which are found in the foods you buy. Here is a quick overview.

Saturated fats are those which solidify at room temperature. They are found in dairy products and meats. They increase the cholesterol level in the body.

Unsaturated fats are liquid at room temperature. They are found in vegetable and seed oils such as safflower, corn and sunflower. They have been shown to lower cholesterol. *But* make certain you purchase *un*refined oils. And keep them refrigerated once they are opened. Refined oils have gone through harsh chemical processes which destroy their beneficial nutrients.

Hydrogenated fats are saturated fats. They are produced by adding hydrogen to unsaturated fats. This process destroys valuable nutrients, such as vitamin E and minerals. You'll want to remove hydrogenated fats from your diet. They are found in many foods such as margarine, snack foods, salad dressings, candy, cakes and breads.

The best solution is to decrease your overall fat intake, and remove hydrogenated fats from your diet.

Enzymes

Enzymes are necessary to regulate every life process. They assist the body in the digestion and assimilation of food, for energy and rebuilding of cells. Enzymes are made up largely of vitamins, minerals and protein compounds.

There are two basic types of enzymes: those manufactured by the body and those occurring in foods. Enzymes are abundant in raw, natural foods such as fresh fruits and vegetables, and raw milk. Cooking can destroy these enzymes, so try to eat at least half of your food raw every day.

Vitamins and Minerals

Vitamins and minerals regulate your metabolism through the enzyme systems. Picture your body as an engine, and the vitamins and minerals as spark plugs. The engine cannot function without them. Both are needed, for vitamins cannot be assimilated without the aid of minerals. The body can manufacture only a few of the vitamins, but the body cannot manufacture any of the minerals. This is why we need both in our food every day.

Best Sources of Vitamins and Minerals

VITAMINS

Vitamins are either water soluble or fat soluble. Vitamin C

and B complex are water soluble. They are absorbed and utilized rapidly, and the excess is quickly excreted. These are not stored in the body so they must be replenished continually during the day. They are more easily destroyed than the fat soluble ones by food processing, cooking and storage. The fat soluble vitamins, A, D, E and K, are first dissolved in fat before absorption and then stored in the body.

Vitamin A	Essential for growth; aids in the formation of teeth and bones, keeps skin and eyes healthy, helps us see at night and builds resistance to respiratory infections. Best sources are carrots, green and yellow fruits and vegetables, fish liver oil, milk and milk products, butter and egg yolks.
B Complex	There is a number of vitamins in this group so we will list them separately. They are necessary for energy, metabolism and muscle tone maintenance.
B^1 (Thiamin)	Necessary for the health of the nerves and blood. Affects carbohydrate metabolism and keeps muscles toned (intestines, heart, stomach). Helps fight motion sickness. Main sources are blackstrap molasses, poultry, brown rice, brewers yeast, whole grains, sunflower seeds, nuts and citrus fruits.
B^2 (Riboflavin)	Helps prevent light-sensitivity of the eyes. Promotes healthy hair, nails and skin. Best sources are cheese, nuts, milk, organ meats, whole grains, broccoli and asparagus.
B^6 (Pyridoxine)	Necessary for fat and protein assimilation. Needed for health of the skin, blood and nerves. Works as a natural diuretic and helps alleviate morning sickness. Main sources are brewers yeast, organ meats, bananas, pea-

nuts, blackstrap molasses, whole grains and green leafy vegetables.

B12
(Cobalamin)

Helps in red blood cell formation and regeneration, promotes growth and increased appetite in children, and maintains a healthy nervous system. Main sources are organ meats, eggs, meat, milk, cheese. Vegetarians who have excluded eggs and dairy products need to take a B12 supplement.

B15
(Pangamic Acid)

Stimulates the glandular and nervous system, and aids fat metabolism. Found in brewers yeast, brown rice, sesame and pumpkin seeds, whole grains.

Biotin

Needed for health of the skin, hair and scalp (helps in prevention of baldness), nerves and mental health. It is needed for fatty-acid production. Found in legumes, nuts, whole grains, fruits and brewers yeast.

Choline

Needed for lecithin formation, liver and gallbladder regulation, fat metabolism. Best sources are green leafy vegetables, legumes, soybeans, egg yolk, organ meats, lecithin.

Folic acid
(B complex)

Essential to blood formation, appetite, body growth and reproduction, hydrochloric-acid formation, and protein metabolism. Best sources are green leafy vegetables, legumes, milk and its products, oysters, salmon, whole grains, nuts and asparagus.

Inositol
(B complex)

Aids in retarding hardening of the arteries, helps lower cholesterol levels, stimulates hair growth, aids in fats metabolism and lecithin formation. Best sources are citrus fruits, nuts, vegetables, whole grains, lecithin, milk, meat, brewers yeast.

Niacin (B complex)	Important for proper functioning of the nervous system. Promotes growth, hydrochloric-acid production, gives healthier-looking skin, reduces cholesterol and aids sex hormone production. Main sources are seafood, milk, poultry, legumes, whole grains, brewers yeast.
Pantothenic acid (B complex)	Necessary for normal digestion and antibody formation. Maintains normal skin, growth and development of central nervous system. Found in legumes, whole grains, nuts, avocado, brewers yeast, organ meats.
PABA (B complex)	Helps give hair its normal color. Needed for blood cell formation and protein metabolism. Keeps skin healthy and smooth. Used in many suntan lotions because it protects against sunburn. Found in liver, brewers yeast, blackstrap molasses, bran, whole grains.
Vitamin C	Also known as ascorbic acid. Essential for general health and growth. Helps wounds to heal and broken bones to mend. Helps fight bacteria and viruses. Strengthens connective tissues and is needed for red blood cell formation. Found largely in citrus fuits, cantaloupe, green peppers, tomatoes, sweet potatoes, strawberries, broccoli, papaya and cauliflower.
Vitamin D (Calciferol)	Works with calcium and phosphorus to build up bones and teeth. Also needed for proper nervous system maintenance. Called the "sunshine" vitamin, for ultraviolet rays from the sun convert a form of cholesterol to vitamin D. Found also in egg yolks, organ meats, fish liver oil, tuna and dairy products.

Vitamin E (Tocopherol)	Very important to the health of the heart. Acts as an antioxidant, suggesting that it may slow the aging process. Important to the health of the reproductive system and all the glands. Helps alleviate fatigue and prevents scar formation internally as well as externally. Main sources are dark leafy vegetables, soybeans, eggs, vegetable oils, almonds, broccoli and wheat germ.
Vitamin F	Necessary for healthy skin, hair and glands. Important in lowering blood cholesterol and combatting heart disease. Found in unrefined vegetable oils (safflower, corn, soy) and sunflower seeds.
Vitamin K	A natural blood-clotting vitamin synthesized within the body. Main sources are green leafy vegetables, alfalfa, cabbage, soybeans, cauliflower, yogurt and egg yolks.

MINERALS

The body needs many different types of minerals, but we are going to touch upon some of the more familiar ones which are necessary for good health and growth. Some of the minerals are needed in large quantities and some (trace minerals) are needed in only minute amounts.

Calcium	More of this mineral exists in your body than any other mineral. You need twice as much calcium as you do phosphorus, for they work in a two-to-one ratio. Calcium builds and maintains bones and teeth, helps blood to clot, regulates heart rhythm; and aids the nervous system. Major sources are milk and dairy products, almonds, dried beans, tofu,

carob, sardines, nuts, sunflower seeds and green vegetables.

Chromium
: Works with insulin in the metabolism of sugar and aids growth. Found in cornmeal, whole wheat, clams, brewers yeast, chicken, corn oil.

Copper
: Aids red blood cell formation, healing processes, hair and skin color. Main sources are legumes, seafood, raisins, bone meal, nuts and molasses.

Iron
: Required for manufacturing of hemoglobin; helps carry oxygen in the blood; promotes stress and disease resistance; helps prevent fatigue. Main sources are brewers yeast, dried fruits, legumes, blackstrap molasses, fish, organ meats, poultry, oatmeal, tomatoes, egg yolks. Iron and calcium deficiencies frequently afflict American woman.

Magnesium
: Necessary for calcium and vitamin C metabolism; essential for normal functioning of nervous and muscular system; needed for blood sugar metabolism (energy). Best sources are apples, bran, soybeans, nuts, figs, lemons, dark green vegetables, whole grains.

Manganese
: Activates various enzymes, also minerals such as calcium and phosphorus. Needed for bone growth and development, reproduction, health of the nerves and vitamin E utilization. Found in bananas, bran, celery, green leafy vegetables, whole grains, nuts, prunes, lettuce and beets.

Phosphorus
: Needed for normal bone and tooth formation. Helps in metabolism of fats and

starches, energy production, and cell growth and repair. Found in fish, eggs, nuts, whole grains, poultry, meat, seeds, raisins, pumpkins.

Potassium   Works with sodium to normalize heart rhythms; necessary for normal muscle tone, nerves and enzyme reaction. Main sources are raisins, peanut butter, oranges, bananas, carrots, apples, seeds, dates, figs, parsley, grapes, seafood, potatoes, tomatoes and peaches.

Selenium   Works with vitamin E in preventing heart attacks, fighting infection, promoting sexual function and as an antioxidant which apparently helps slow aging. Found in bran, onions, tomatoes, garlic, asparagus, tuna, brewers yeast.

Sodium   Needed for proper muscle contraction and nerve function, regulates normal cellular fluid level. Found in cheese, milk, seafood, carrots, beets, celery, prunes, oatmeal, spinach.

Sulfur   Purifies and cleanses the blood. Essential for health of the hair, skin and nails. Found in bran, eggs, nuts, fish, cheese, cabbage, apples, onions, peas.

Zinc   Helps direct the whole enzyme system. Essential to the health of the skin, prostate gland and all glands. Necessary for operation of the muscles, health of all blood vessels. Aids burn and wound healing. Found in brewers yeast, seafood, soybeans, spinach, nuts and seeds, whole grains and eggs.

Water

About two-thirds of your body is water. You can survive

without food for weeks, but without water, only three or four days. Water regulates your body temperature, acts as a lubricant, collects waste products from cells, aids in tissue growth, aids the metabolism of nutrients, plays a role in bio-chemical reactions, and flushes toxins from the body.

Fruits and vegetables contain water but not enough to meet your daily requirements. We recommend that you consume from seven to eight glasses of water each day, in addition to the fruits and vegetables you eat. We note sadly that many people drink barely any water, or fresh fruit or vegetables juices each day. Some people tell us that it's hard to drink a glass of water, especially when they aren't thirsty. We tell them to squeeze a bit of lemon or lime in the water to add a tangy taste—plus vitamin C. We also tell them not to try to drink it all at once. They should fill up a glass and simply sip on it. When it's empty, they can fill it up again and sip some more. Before the day is over, they will have consumed the required amount of water.

There was a time when all water was clean and unpolluted. Unfortunately, today clean water is a rarity. Often what comes out of our tap tastes so horrible and contains such harmful ingredients that many people, such as we, are turning to bottled water. Some tap water has such a high level of sodium that bottled water is a necessity.

We recommend you look into purchasing bottled water. You can purchase it at your grocery store as well as at a health food store. It usually comes in one-gallon containers. Or, you can have bottled water delivered in a five-gallon container to your home. The supplier will provide you an easy-to-use dispenser stand, also. We keep our bottled water in our kitchen and use it for both drinking and cooking.

Bottled water can be either spring water or distilled water.

Spring water is unpolluted water which has bubbled up from deep underground. Spring water contains many natural minerals.

Distilled water, some people feel, is the best water to drink, since it is the most pure. If you drink it, we recommend that you take a mineral supplement, because distilled water contains no minerals. You can purchase this water or buy a distiller that will distill your own tap water for only the cost of the electricity it uses.

Working Together

All of the above nutrients must work together in a proper balance to furnish you with good health. You need to make sure your food is of the highest quality so that you can be supplied with all the needed components.

All the essentials for good health are available to us, but the typical American's diet supplies the bodies with poor quality foods. One of the reasons is the crazy pace of life that so many people get trapped in. People tend to rely on convenience, pre-packaged foods—foods that have been processed and refined, thus devoid of most, if not all, of the vitamins, minerals, enzymes, fiber and trace minerals. Quite often, chemical additives "replace" these lost nutrients. The foods bear little resemblance to the foods as God had given them, and of course they are sorely lacking in the nutrients necessary for a healthy, energy-filled life. They are foods that will satisfy your taste and fill you up, but they will not feed your body.

To show how the American diet has changed, let's look at this comparative study published in *U.S. News and World Report* (Dec. 8, 1980).

What is eaten in the diet	1979 (per person)	Change since 1960	
Soft drinks	37.5 gallons	Up	175.7%
Poultry	61.6 pounds	Up	79.1%
Cheese	22.4 pounds	Up	71.0%
Processed vegetables	65.0 pounds	Up	29.0%
Fish	17.6 pounds	Up	28.5%
Fats, oils, including butter and margarine	61.2 pounds	Up	26.2%

Sugar, sweeteners	137.0	pounds	Up	26.2%
Beef	79.6	pounds	Up	23.8%
Processed fruit	58.0	pounds	Up	15.3%
Pork	65.0	pounds	Up	7.8%
Refined flour, cereal products	150.0	pounds	Up	2.0%
Fresh vegetables	144.3	pounds	Down	1.2%
Fresh fruit	81.3	pounds	Down	9.7%
Milk, cream	32.9	gallons	Down	12.4%
Eggs	274		Down	15.4%

Many of the "Downs" should be up and some of the "Ups" should be down. Americans are switching from healthy foods to foods that are non-nutritive, hence the problem of over-weight and under-nourished people in our country.

In our next chapter we'll be giving you a healthy eating plan. *Moderation* is a word to keep in mind as you read that chapter. It's a human tendency to overdo in many areas of life. For example, instead of consuming a few pounds of sugar a year, people are consuming huge amounts. They then switch to honey, but continue to consume huge amounts. Excessive-ness can cause us problems. Use moderation.

Another word to keep in mind, throughout your life and as you finish this book, is *gradual.* If you are going to change your exercise or eating, it should be a gradual process. If you faithfully persist, you'll be able to reflect back and see that you've made great progress. It's not the crazy blitz, but steady progress, that shows lasting results.

If you've read this far in *Free To Be Fit,* you probably care about your health. Unfortunately many people don't start really caring until something goes wrong. Our purpose is to show you a way to have an energy-filled, vibrant life that you can give to our Lord. In John 10:10 we read, "The thief comes only to steal, to kill, to destroy; I have come that men may have life, and may have it in all its fullness" (NEB). God wants you to be healthy—in *all* areas of your life. And He wants you to do something about it *before* trouble strikes.

We want you to consider the foods as *God* put them on this earth for our nourishment and enjoyment. These are the same foods that our ancestors ate. Only during the last 25 to 30 years has food begun to suffer the indignities of commercial processing.

As you continue reading this book, ask the Holy Spirit for guidance and wisdom, that you might choose foods that will glorify Him in your body. He will show you.

We'll do our part to help you, also.

"So whether you eat or drink or whatever you do, do it all for the glory of God" (1 Cor. 10:31, NIV).

Chapter Nine

REAL FOODS FOR REAL FITNESS

   The eating plan we are going to suggest for you is not highly restrictive. It is restrictive about sugar, white flours, salt and hydrogenated fats, plus processed and refined foods. But we want you to eat a wide variety of foods—natural foods. As we have continually stressed, these are the foods that God put on this earth that we might enjoy eating *and* maintain good health so we can function for His glory.
   Your body will function best if you feed it a balance of proper foods. Its functioning will improve with regular exercise, proper rest (sleep *and* relaxation), and most importantly, a solid, Christ-centered spiritual life.
   We will first discuss the foods you should definitely avoid.

FOODS TO AVOID

Refined Sugar and Sugar-Laden Products

   Sugar does not contain any nutrients, only calories. In fact, it robs your body's supply of nutrients, especially vitamin B. It has been shown to contribute to diabetes, low blood sugar, heart disease, obesity (the sugar is stored as fat), peptic ulcers and tooth decay. Only 100 years ago the average person consumed 20 pounds of sugar per year. Now the average person consumes 120-140 pounds per year. That is over 500 calories worth of sugar a day.
   Sugar is found in nearly all the foods you can buy. It has been estimated that 92% of foods found in the supermarket

contain sugar. As you read package labels, look for the following: brown sugar, powdered sugar, corn syrup or corn sweeteners, dextrose, maltose, glucose, invert sugar, sorbital, levu-
lose, turbinado sugar, clean raw sugar, sucrose, fructose,
artificial sweeteners.

Some of the foods that contain large amounts of sugar
are: jams and jellies, ice cream, gelatin, cakes, candy, cookies,
soft drinks, ketchup (29%), salad dressings (30%), Hamburger
Helper (23%), bouillon cubes (15%), canned vegetables (11%),
whipped toppings (65%).

White Flour and Products Made with White Flour

White flour has gone through a refining process which removes the germ and bran. That refining removes nearly all the
nutrients from the flour and leaves the endosperm, which is
mostly starch, and a small amount of poor quality protein.

On package labels, white flour may also be listed as en-
riched, unbleached, self-rising, all-purpose, instantized or cake
flour.

White flour can be found in bread, biscuits, noodles, pan-
cakes, waffles, crackers, pastas, pies, pastries, cakes, cookies,
and baking mixes.

Hydrogenated Fats

Margarine is an *artificial* food which has been stripped of
nutrients and embellished with artificial color and flavor, preservatives and vitamin A.

Other hydrogenated fats are hydrogenated oils, hydrogenated peanut butter, vegetable shortening and any products
that contain hydrogenated or partially-hydrogenated fats.

Presweetened Cereals

Many of these are full of sugar. Here are some examples:

Grape Nuts (6.6%), Raisin Bran (10.6%), All Bran (20%), Alpha Bits (40%), Cap'n Crunch (43%), Apple Jacks (55%), Sugar Smacks (61.3%).

Fried Foods

Foods prepared in this manner are usually saturated with fat. They are high in poor-quality calories and are harder to digest than non-fried foods.

Smoked or Processed Meats

Ham, bacon, sausage, luncheon meats, hot dogs, salami, bologna, corned beef and pastrami all come under this category. Most of them contain great amounts of saturated fat.

Refined Grains

White rice, bolted and degermed cornmeal, and others suffer from the same malady as white flour; all the "good stuff" has been stripped away.

Coffee, Tea, Soft Drinks and Chocolate

All of these items contain caffeine, which acts as a stimulant to the body's system. It also irritates the kidneys, bladder and stomach. You can develop an addiction to caffeine which will cause you to crave even more. If you quit the habit, you will experience withdrawal symptoms, including headaches, jitters, and nausea.

All soft drinks also consist of chemicals, water, and sugar or artificial sweeteners (derived from coal tar). They contain no food value. They fill you up without feeding your body, and thus take the place of nourishing food.

If you begin to avoid the above-mentioned foods, you are already on your way to better health.

There are also some foods which you should cut back on. As we wrote earlier, moderation is an important key to proper eating and fitness.

FOODS TO CUT BACK ON

Salt

Most people are consuming ten to twenty times more salt than is needed in their diet. This large amount is contributing to hypertension. It has been estimated that about 60 million people in the U.S. have some form of high blood pressure. Hypertension contributes to over half of the deaths every year in the U.S., and many people unknowingly suffer from some form of it. They don't find out until struck with a heart attack or a stroke. Salt also contributes to kidney distress and edema (water retention).

Don't use salt at the table or add it while cooking. Just like sugar, it is in many of our foods. A dish of cottage cheese can have more salt than a handful of salted potato chips! Look on the labels for salt, MSG, brine, sodium. You will find sodium derivatives used often as preservatives within your foods.

Avoid all highly salted foods, such as salted nuts, pretzels, crackers, potato chips, pickles, olives, Worcestershire sauce, fast foods, processed foods, luncheon meats. (Most of these items can be purchased in unsalted forms.)

Saturated Fats

Saturated fats are found in meat and dairy products, as well as in three plant products: coconut oil, palm kernel oil and cocoa butter. You will find these plant products in many bakery items.

FOODS TO INCLUDE IN YOUR DIET

1. PROTEIN
   Animal:
   Beef, lean: eat only two or three times weekly. Chicken or turkey: remove the skin before eating. Fish: prefer the less fatty types. Eggs.
   Vegetable:
   Dried beans and peas, lentils, grains, seeds and nuts, nut butters

2. DAIRY PRODUCTS
   Raw certified milk or non-instant dry milk powder
   Yogurt, kefir, acidophilus milk
   Cottage cheese, pot or farmers cheese, ricotta cheese
   Cream cheese
   Cheese (uncolored)
   Buttermilk

3. VEGETABLES
   Eat a great many of them raw and with the skins intact. (This is only a partial list.)

artichokes	eggplant	potatoes
asparagus	green peppers	pumpkin
beans	Jerusalem	rhubarb
beets and	artichokes	rutabagas
greens	kale	spinach
broccoli	kohlrabi	sprouts
brussel sprouts	lettuce	summer squash
cabbage	mushrooms	sweet potatoes
carrots	mustard greens	tomatoes
cauliflower	okra	turnips and
celery	onions	greens
collard greens	parsley	winter squash
corn	parsnips	yams
cucumbers	peas	zucchini

4. FRUITS
   Eat as many as you can with skins intact. (This is just a
   partial list of the different fruits available to you.)

apples	melons
bananas	oranges
blackberries	papaya
blueberries	peaches
cranberries	pears
grapefruit	pineapples
grapes	strawberries
dried fruits (in moderation)	lemons and limes

5. WHOLE GRAINS
   Breads and Flours

Pumpernickel bread	Corn flour
Corn bread	Brown rice flour
Rye bread	Whole wheat (100%
Tortillas (whole wheat or	whole wheat)
corn)	Pita or pocket bread
Whole wheat flour or 100%	(100% whole wheat)
stone-ground whole	Muffins, bagels,
wheat flour	crackers (all from
Soy flour	whole grain flours
Rye flour	only)

Pasta and Grains
Macaroni, spaghetti, lasagne, noodles (all can be purchased with whole wheat, spinach, sesame, artichoke or
vegetable flavor).

Brown rice	Millet
Buckwheat	Bulgur wheat
Bran	Cornmeal (white or
Wild rice	yellow)
Oats (rolled or steel cut)	Barley

Cereals
Whole grains: any of the above-mentioned grains (singly or in combination) can be cooked and used as a cereal.
Rolled oats, wheat flakes or rye flakes (used either as a cold or hot cereal).
Breakfast cereals made from wheat, rice or oats (as long as they are not coated with sugar or honey).
Shredded wheat, Wheatena, Zoom, Cream of Rye
Seven- or nine-grain cereals

6. BEVERAGES
   Cereal grain beverages: Caffix, Pero, Postum, Heritage (use as coffee substitutes)
   Herb teas
   Fruit juices (unsweetened)
   Vegetable juices
   Mineral water (Perrier is a low-sodium brand)

7. SWEETENERS
   Raw, unfiltered honey, molasses (blackstrap or unsulfured). Use sparingly.
   Apple or other fruit concentrates
   Dried fruit
   Carob powder

8. FATS
   Use moderate amounts of fats and oils.
   Butter (sweet cream, unsalted)
   Oils (unrefined): sunflower, safflower (best all-around oil), peanut, soy, sesame seed, olive, corn

9. SEASONINGS
   Vegetable seasoning (Vegit by Gaylord Hauser is recommended.)
   Assorted herbs and spices
   Vegetable broth (Bernard Jensen's brand is recommended.)

Cider vinegar
Ketchup (sweetened with honey)
Mayonnaise (sweetened with honey) (Hains is an excellent brand.)
Mustard (stone-ground)

10. SNACKS
Popcorn
Various nuts: peanuts, walnuts, almonds, cashews, pecans, brazil nuts, etc.
Various seeds; sesame seeds, sunflower seeds, pumpkin seeds, etc.
(When using seeds or nuts, remember to buy *raw, unsalted* ones.)
Raw vegetables and fresh fruit
Peanut butter and celery
Whole grain crackers with cheese
Frozen grapes, cherries, pineapple chunks or bananas

A RECOMMENDED DAILY MENU

BREAKFAST	EXAMPLE
Fruit or fruit juice	Sliced peaches
Main dish	Whole grain cereal served with yogurt or milk
Bread	Bran muffin

LUNCH	
Main dish	Tuna salad on Pita bread
Vegetable and/or salad	Marinated raw vegetable on bed of sprouts
Bread or grains	(Pita bread in the main course)
Fruit	Apple

DINNER

Main dish	Sesame-baked chicken
Vegetable	Green beans and yellow squash with sliced almonds
Salad	Spinach salad with oil dressing
Potato, grain dish or pasta	Barley and rice pilaf
Bread (optional)	Whole wheat roll

DESSERTS

Fresh fruits, puddings and custards
Periodically you can incorporate cookies, cakes, pies, etc. But try to bake them with ingredients that are on the "Foods to Include" list.

DAILY GUIDELINES

1. *Protein.* Eat two servings a day and concentrate on chicken, fish and vegetable proteins. Don't forget eggs.

2. *Dairy products.* Eat one to two servings a day with concentration on cultured milk products such as yogurt, kefir and acidophilus milk—they are easy to digest. We do not feel adults need to drink milk every day to stay healthy. When using milk, use *raw, certified* milk, if possible. Pasteurized, homogenized milk has been shown to be very hard to digest for many people; and pasteurization destroys many valuable nutrients. We also suggest the *non-instant* milk powder, which has not undergone a high heat process. We prefer to get our dairy products by using them in recipes.

3. *Vegetables.* Eat a variety of many vegetables (raw or lightly cooked) during the day. Make sure you include at least one leafy green and one yellow vegetable in your day's meal plan.

Also eat at least two raw vegetable salads with an unrefined oil dressing.

4. *Sprouts.* Include one to two servings of these daily, especially during the winter months. You can use them in salads, on sandwiches, in bread, and in many other foods.

5. *Fruits.* Eat a variety every day and make sure you include at least one citrus. Juices are great but not as a substitute for eating the whole fruit. Chewing keeps your teeth and gums in good condition, and whole fruit is full of fiber.

6. *Whole grains.* Eat four or more servings a day in the form of whole grain breads and cereals, in sprouted form, or in side dishes and pastas.

7. *Beverages.* Drink plenty of liquids during the day, especially water. We, of course, recommend either spring or distilled water. We add a squeeze of lime or lemon to the water for flavor. Six to eight glasses of water a day is a good goal.

8. *Fats.* Use at least one tablespoon of oil a day, as it is a good source of essential fatty acids. It is necessary even if you are trying to lose weight. Make sure it comprises no more than 15% to 20% of your daily calorie intake.

9. *Raw food.* Eat at least 50% of each meal uncooked. Cooking breaks down fiber and can destroy many nutrients.

10. *Moderate servings.* Even people who are not overweight can tend to overeat and thus feel stuffed after their meal. Leave the table feeling that you could have eaten a little more. This is the *secret* to weight loss, as well as good health.

11. *Mealtime beverages.* Don't drink liquids with your meals, for they will dilute your digestive juices and thus hamper digestion. If you are very thirsty, drink half an hour before the meal—lots of water. The water will pass through and won't stifle your appetite, but it will quench your desire for water or liquids. If you must drink something with the meal, just *sip* your beverage. By sipping, you will find you won't consume as much.

12. *Chewing.* Chew until the food is mulch. This will enhance digestion and assimilation of the food. Remember, your

stomach does not have any teeth! Also, by chewing the food well, you will be satisfied with less food, hence, fewer calories.

13. *Variety.* No one food can supply all the nutrients you need. Most people eat a very limited diet, especially in the realm of vegetables. Our list of vegetables proves that there is a wide variety available. Also, by eating a varied diet, you can help prevent certain food allergies. Doctors are finding that a lot of the foods which people are allergic to are ones that are heavily consumed, such as wheat and corn.

14. *Desserts.* Cookies, cakes, pies, etc., are not bad if you make them with whole grains and natural sweeteners. Don't make them a daily occurrence, however. Eat more fresh fruit as dessert.

15. *Dinner.* Eat bigger breakfasts and lunches and lighter dinners.

16. *EXERCISE!*

Additional Weight-Loss Guidelines

1. Limit portion sizes. You need to eat a wide variety of foods, but just don't eat large portions of them. You do not need as much food as you think you do.

2. Nuts have been listed as possible snacks, but eat only a few, as they are very high in fat. Instead of wolfing a large fist, just munch on a couple of them, and make sure you chew them well.

3. When you eat dairy products, concentrate on low fat ones. And don't indulge in too much cheese.

4. If you sauté food, do it in broth or vegetable juice rather than in fat.

5. Eat bread during breakfast and lunch, but don't have any at dinner.

CONSERVING FOOD NUTRIENTS

1. Eat mostly fresh fruits and vegetables, rather than fro-

zen or canned ones. The fresher the produce the higher the nutritional value.

2. Don't buy bruised, injured or wilted produce. Blemishes indicate that it could be old, which means it has lost valuable nutrients. Buy produce that looks fresh and bright in color.

3. Don't buy too much produce, as the nutritional value decreases each day of storage.

4. When preparing produce, wash it quickly in cold water just before you're ready to use it. Never wash it before then. Never soak the produce.

5. If preparing vegetables by slicing or chopping, do it just before using. And if they have not been sprayed with toxic insecticides, do not peel them. Many valuable nutrients and fiber lie in the skin, as well as just beneath it.

6. Meats, if frozen, should be cooked without thawing so as to prevent losses of B vitamins and minerals. Oven cooking and broiling are the best methods for retaining the nutrients.

7. Losses in nutrients in produce are accelerated by heat, air and baking soda. Don't add baking soda to vegetables being cooked.

8. The best methods for cooking produce are steaming, baking or stir frying. *Don't boil vegetables.* In just four minutes of boiling, 20% to 45% of the nutrients go into the water.

9. Undercook the vegetables, for they will continue to cook even after they have been removed from the heat.

10. Don't reheat your vegetable leftovers. Serve them in a cold salad.

11. Don't thaw frozen vegetables before cooking. Make sure your freezer's temperature is kept at 0° Fahrenheit in order to retain the nutrients.

EATING OUT

The question we most frequently get when we give our seminar is, "Can't I eat out anymore?"

Of course you can. Just follow your food plan and choose

the foods that best fit into it. We eat out often and have no problem.

For example, order a big salad or go to a restaurant that has a good salad bar. Watch the dressing, though; most dressings are full of sugar. We often bring our own small container of homemade dressing, or, we order lemon slices for our salad.

Order chicken or fish, broiled, and tell them to hold the salt. Stay away from soups, since they are usually loaded with salt. We usually order a baked potato as our vegetable. If the bread served is white, shun it, but if you're served dark bread, which many places are doing, go ahead and partake.

Dessert? You really don't *need* it, do you? But if you just *have* to have a dessert, order fruit!

DEDICATION DEMANDS DISCIPLINE

We're confident that if you study and apply the information given in this chapter, your state of health will head upwards. Try to follow our health program as much as possible, but don't be legalistic; you can make a few allowances *periodically* (not regularly). Remember, you are not under the law. You are under grace.

For example, if you go to a restaurant to eat Mexican food, but you're served white flour tortillas, don't be a martyr and refuse. Eat them. You'll live.

Simply try to eat and exercise properly wherever you are and whenever you can. If you "blow it," don't worry or do penance. Realize you did wrong, forgive yourself and forget it. Press ahead. If you are dedicated to changing your eating habits, remember that DEDICATION DEMANDS DISCIPLINE.

It's up to you. We're with you. So is the Lord!

". . . forgetting those things which are behind, and reaching forth unto those things which are before, I press toward the mark for the prize of the high calling of God in Christ Jesus" (Phil. 3:13-14, KJV).

Chapter Ten

MANAGING STRESS

Recently we were shocked by the sudden death of a close friend. Bill had just finished a regular weekend tennis game when he collapsed in the club locker room and died.

Bill, in his 40's, was no obvious candidate for early death. His weight was normal. He played tennis in most of the club tournaments. He avoided alcohol and tobacco. Why, then, such an untimely death?

Bill's job may have to take the blame. Recently made a dean at the local university, Bill inherited problems for which he had no previous training or experience. Under the pressures of declining enrollments, budget reductions, and faculty demands for salary increases, Bill found himself caught between the concerns of his former faculty colleagues and the administrative realities of his new job. Moreover, the new responsibilities left little time for the research and writing projects he had nurtured for years.

In short, Bill was a victim of stress. The pressures and demands normally associated with modern corporate and business life had reached into the apparently serene offices of the academic establishment and claimed another victim.

Stress and its insidious effects is receiving a lot of attention these days from psychologists, psychiatrists and physicians. A considerable number of articles on stress have appeared in popular magazines. And the professionals are cranking out an expanding volume of literature that both sounds the alarm and suggests solutions.

Psychiatrists and psychologists divide stress problems into various categories. Some is called "real" stress—that is, stress produced by some event, such as an automobile accident. But there is also stress which is "imagined"—stress produced by suspicions, fears, and anxieties.

Also the psychiatrists speak of "episodic" stress over against "chronic" stress. Episodic stress is that which occurs for a short time and then disappears. Moving to a new city, taking a new job, preparing for an examination—all may bring on episodic stress. Chronic stress situations differ. These include problems over which people feel they have little or no control. The hustle, bustle, noise, pollution and dangers of modern city life produce stress for many people. These are constant problems and dangers that no single person can do anything about. This sort of stress, many psychiatrists insist, modern people must learn to cope with.

Medical experts are concerned about the physical reactions to stress. There are measurable increases in heartbeat, respiration and the level of blood sugar when stress occurs. The pupils dilate, muscles tense, and digestion slows. The body exhibits a "fight or flight" response normally associated with physical danger. The body unconsciously prepares to resist or to flee. The physical response is automatic.

It is important to consider the stressful situation in your own life. A helpful tool for such consideration is the Holmes/ Rahe Social Readjustment Rating Scale. It provides a list of events which might be having an impact upon your life, and which could be a source of stress. The chart provides a way to locate forms of stress which might push you toward serious trouble.

On the chart, circle "yes" or "no" for each event that has occurred in your life during the last year or that you anticipate happening in the near future. Then go back over the chart and circle the intensity point value of each "yes" answer. Add up the total points. The higher the total, the greater your chances are of being under stress which could result in illness. In general, people who score between 150 and 300 have one chance in two of developing a serious stress-related illness. People scoring 150 and below have about one chance in three of illness occurring.

STRESS-RATING SCALE

Event	Answer		Point Value
Death of spouse	Yes	No	100
Divorce	Yes	No	73
Marriage separation	Yes	No	65
Jail term	Yes	No	63
Death in family	Yes	No	63
Personal injury or illness	Yes	No	53
Marriage	Yes	No	50
Fired from work	Yes	No	47
Marital reconciliation	Yes	No	45
Retirement	Yes	No	45
Change in family member's health	Yes	No	44
Pregnancy	Yes	No	40
Sex difficulties	Yes	No	39
Addition to family	Yes	No	39
Business readjustment	Yes	No	39
Change in financial status	Yes	No	38
Death of a close friend	Yes	No	37
Change to different field of work	Yes	No	36
Change in number of arguments in marriage	Yes	No	36
Loan or mortgage over $10,000	Yes	No	30
Foreclosure of loan or mortgage	Yes	No	30
Change in work responsibilities	Yes	No	29
Son or daughter leaving home	Yes	No	29
In-law problems	Yes	No	29
Outstanding personal achievement	Yes	No	28
Spouse stops or begins work	Yes	No	26
Completing or starting school	Yes	No	26

Change in living conditions	Yes	No	25
Trouble with your boss	Yes	No	23
Change in work hours, conditions	Yes	No	20
Change in residence	Yes	No	20
Change in recreational habits	Yes	No	19
Change in church activities	Yes	No	19
Change in social activities	Yes	No	18
Loan or mortgage under $10,000	Yes	No	17
Change in sleeping habits	Yes	No	16
Change in number of family gatherings	Yes	No	15
Change in eating habits	Yes	No	15
Vacation	Yes	No	13
Christmas season	Yes	No	12
Minor violation of the law	Yes	No	11

Keep in mind that the stress chart serves as a means of prediction only. You may score high but not get sick. On the other hand, remember that the chart has been used successfully to predict trouble for enough people to give it significant credibility in medical circles.

Techniques for Stress Management

If you scored high on the stress chart, you need to examine your life and try to find out which stress-producing events or conditions are under your control. Once you begin doing this, you will discover something quite interesting: many events that cause the most difficulty are simply outside of any one person's control. Once you reach this discovery, you can begin to see how important both exercise *and* active faith are to a person's health.

It is important to remember that stress itself is neutral, both morally and physically. It is neither good nor bad. It is triggered sometimes by positive situations and sometimes by negative situations. A new job, new responsibilities, confrontation with new or confusing cultural situations all cause stress. And sometimes it is stress which helps a person to perform at his optimum efficiency and ability. For example, an athlete is only as good as his competition makes him. And we are only as good as the stress we experience makes us.

Yet we would be remiss if we did not point out some other factors concerning stress. Often it is stress which can drive us to God and to doing something about ourselves which we would not otherwise do.

We mentioned earlier that the professional literature about stress is increasing. More and more people point to the stress of modern life which is the cause of more and more problems, physical and mental. Yet all reach the conclusion that stress is a natural part of the human condition. It is here, it is inevitable, it is part of life. And if it is all of these things, it, too, is something that is here in order to drive us to God.

An analysis of stressful conditions suggests that stress can be divided into two types: objectifiable stress situations and nonobjectifiable stress situations. The objectifiable stress situations are those which can be identified, located, analyzed, considered and, to some extent, resolved by some specific measures or treatment. You can change jobs (if your work situation is the problem), you can buy a new car (if breakdowns are bothering you), you can avoid certain people (if they create problems), you can negotiate another loan (if finances are troubling you). However difficult any of these things might be to do (and none of them may be easy), at least there is *something* you can do. There is an objectifiable problem out there which is bugging you. And your task is to find it, examine it, and set about resolving it.

But the other kind of stress, more troubling, is the kind of stress which is ultimately nonobjectifiable in origin. This is the stress that people must learn to live with, because there is no single object or thing out there producing the stressful situations and conditions. And since there is no object, no specific thing or person, there is nothing which can be isolated, controlled, eliminated or changed. There are countless examples of how this sort of stress affects people: pressure to perform beyond one's personal sense of capability; inner dissatisfaction or frustration with one's self; a sense of inadequacy, incompetence, guilt or worthlessness.

There is nothing odd about these feelings or stresses. In fact, to experience such stress is to indicate a sensitivity to the reality of human existence. After all, stress as a "free-floating anxiety" which remains unattached to any specific thing or situation is common to all human lives. When we consider that we never chose to be born into this world, we never chose the time or conditions of our birth, we never chose our parents, we never chose our native intelligence, we never chose the advantages or limitations of the financial conditions of our family, then we experience what some thinkers have termed the "thrownness" of human life. We feel threatened by the fact that we seem to have been randomly thrown into a world which is not of our own making and over which we have little or no control. Moreover, we are confronted daily with the sense that much of what we must do to survive in this world does nothing to help solve the many really important problems that face mankind. What significance does trudging to the office, the classroom, to the hospital or clinic, or driving a truck or taxi have in the face of pollution, starvation, threat of nuclear war, soaring crime rates, and drugs in the local high school?

Questions about the meaningfulness and significance of one's own occupation and preoccupations, in the face of serious worldwide problems, produce for many people an uncomfortable sense that things are wrong, that human life is out of joint, that much of what is being done in the world is irrelevant to what is really important. Yet the sense of responsibility, coupled with blame, guilt, hopelessness, and impotence accompany such insights and compound the problem.

But how can such feelings be relieved? What concrete, specific things can anyone do to change these stressful conditions? Certainly we cannot, as Nicodemus told Jesus, return to be reborn in different circumstances.

Yet the feelings of worthlessness, failure, anxiousness and

doubt continue to produce this nonobjectifiable, uncontrollable stress. The stress appears because a person is aware of legitimate questions which have bothered philosophers, theologians, preachers and saints for centuries. Yet some people react to this sort of stress with self-destructive measures— alcohol, smoking, overeating, physical violence, temper tantrums, irritability, distress. Most of the time they are unaware of why they react these ways. They are simply uncomfortable, troubled, unbalanced, alienated from themselves, from God, and from other people.

But what is the real solution? It must first of all be spiritual. If we believe that God created us, that He has a plan for our lives, that harmony with His plan for us is possible, and that we can commit ourselves to His will in the world, then we can rest. Rest requires faith, trust. Faith casts care, worry, anxiety upon God who loves us and cares for us. Remember Isaiah 26:3: "Thou wilt keep him in perfect peace whose mind is stayed on thee: because he trusteth in thee" (KJV). And recall with us the words Jesus gave His disciples:

"Let not your heart be troubled, trust in God; trust also in me. . . . I will not leave you as orphans; I will come to you. . . . Peace I leave with you; my peace I give to you. . . . Do not let your hearts be troubled, and do not be fearful" (John 14:1, 18, 27, NIV).

Read the Scriptures and discover that Jesus knows all about stress, worry, anxiety. And He gave the solution—*trust* in Him.

Yet we also know that "faith without works is dead." There is some work to do in order to restore the body which has been assaulted daily by stress. The ravages of stress have caused for you and others immeasureable damage to the body, the temple of God. The constant barrage of pressures, responsibilities, frustrations, failures, questions and contradictions bring the physical consequences identified earlier as the symptoms of stress.

To work out your faith, you must first make a daily habit of reading the Scriptures, a thoughtful and quiet time devoted o meditation on the Word and fellowship with the Lord in prayer. Then comes your program of vigorous exercise.

We believe, and our lives and the lives of others prove, that a program of this sort is the only proper solution to the stress-ful conditions of modern life. God made this world we live in, He put us here, He has a way for us to live, and He arranges the conditions and circumstances to drive us to trust in Him. Only when your life is under God's control can you be *free to be fit.*

"But blessed is the man who trusts in the Lord, whose confidence is in him. He will be like a tree planted by the water that sends out its roots by the stream. It does not fear when heat comes; its leaves are always green. It has no worries in a year of drought and never fails to bear fruit" (Jer. 17:7-8, NIV).

Appendix

JOGGING/RUNNING

Recently the President's Council on Physical Fitness and Sports published a list of popular forms of exercise. The list rated each in terms of how much it would help cardio-respiratory (heart and lungs) endurance, muscular endurance, muscular strength, flexibility, balance and general well-being. Many people were surprised to see that running had been ranked the highest in nearly every category. And running emerged with the highest total score.

Physical fitness	Running	Bicycling	Swimming	Handball	Tennis	Walking	Golf	Bowling
Cardio-respiratory								
endurance	21	19	21	19	16	13	8	5
Muscular endurance	20	18	20	18	16	14	8	5
Muscular strength	17	16	14	15	14	11	9	5
Flexibility	9	9	15	16	14	7	8	7
Balance	17	18	12	17	16	8	8	6
General well-being								
Weight control	21	20	15	19	16	13	6	5
Muscle definition	14	15	14	11	13	11	7	7
Digestion	13	12	13	13	12	11	7	7
Sleep	16	15	16	12	11	14	6	6
Total	148	142	140	140	128	102	66	51

Almost all of the data available indicates that if you were to limit yourself to one form of exercise, running or jogging would be the best one to choose. It's true that your upper body gets little exercise when jogging. But from a physical fitness stand-point, jogging does more for general conditioning and the pro-longation of life than any other single form of exercise.

Getting Started

Getting started is probably the most difficult aspect of jog-ging. After all, it's easy to read about, easy to think about, but difficult to begin doing. Often it helps to find a friend who would like to jog with you. You won't feel quite so conspicuous out on the streets in your shorts or sweats if someone is beside you.

But jogging is important enough to your health to take precedence over shyness. So find a regular time to dress, warm up, jog and shower. The decision to find the time indi-cates that you are on the way. And if you hesitate to be seen shuffling along in your present physical condition, jog early in the morning or late at night when few people are likely to be about to see you.

The best way to begin a jogging program is the walk-run. Begin by walking at a quick-step for 10 minutes. After 10 min-utes, stop and check your heart rate by pressing two fingers on the inside of your arm just above the wrist, or just behind your "Adam's apple" on your neck. Your PR should not be as high as 70% of your maximum yet. But your heart should be beating considerably more than its normal PR.

The fast walk will gradually strengthen your heart and your legs. Next combine walking with brief spurts of jogging. After a few weeks you will be able to complete successully and without strain the entire 10 minutes without walking at all. And the more you jog, the stronger you will get.

At the point when you can jog easily for 10 or 20 minutes,

occasionally check your pulse rate while at rest during the day. You will find that your heartbeat is much slower than it used to be. There may be actually 20 fewer beats per minute than before you started jogging. And this can total as many as 20,000 to 30,000 fewer beats per day. At the same time your lungs have become conditioned to process more air with less effort. And the number and size of blood vessels are increasing. The conditioning is also enhancing muscle tone while reducing blood pressure. That is total fitness!

When you first begin to jog, you may experience some stiffness in your muscles and joints. That is good. If you don't feel some discomfort at first, it means you are not working hard enough. Stiffness, then, is a *good* sign.

The best solution for easing the stiffness and soreness that accompanies jogging is to stretch before *and* after you do your workout. Simple exercises such as bending ten to twenty times, trunk twisters and jumping jacks relieve and prevent strains. Discover your own loosening-up routine. In time your own series of stretches that work best for you will become a regular part of your jogging.

Shoes

The most important equipment for jogging is a *good* pair of shoes. There are many brand names and styles available, ranging in price from $10 to $90. Remember bona-fide brands and counterfeits are not always easily distinguished by the novice; cheap copies of the best running shoes abound. When buying footwear, be willing to pay for quality. Proper shoes are important, since the pounding of your feet on pavement can cause serious discomfort and damage to ankles, knees, hips and back. Don't make your initial run wearing a $4.95 discount store bargain. Your body will never forgive you!

Please note that an athletic shoe is designed for a particular activity and surface. A racquetball, tennis, or basketball shoe is designed for quick stopping and starting, and is rein-

forced for lateral movement and strain. A jogging shoe, however, must have a certain degree of roundness on the heels
and toes to help provide a fluid motion when running in a single direction. Should you attempt to run in a basketball or racquetball shoe, you will find that your foot slaps the ground
awkwardly. You will have to adjust your running style to the
shoe, and soon you'll be running improperly. That could lead
to injury.

Jogging Surfaces

The surface upon which you are going to jog is important,
too. A good surface for jogging is one which allows some give
as your feet strike it. A poor surface is one what is so hard and
unyielding that you can experience discomfort and pain from
the ankle all the way to the lower back.

The following chart lists various surfaces for jogging and
their relative quality, as well as where you might find them.

Surface	Rating	Location
1. Sand	Good	Beaches, some country roads
2. Grass	Good	Parks, schools
3. Tarton	Average	Universities/Colleges
4. Gravel	Fair	High schools, country roads
5. Dirt	Fair/Poor	Country roads
6. Asphalt	Poor	City streets/roads
7. Concrete	Poor	City sidewalks

Generally, the more give a surface has, the less pressure
you exert on the joints of your hips, knees, and ankles. If you
cannot find a good jogging surface, be sure you are using a
shoe with plenty of padding. You may even want to add some
additional cushioning (check with a sporting goods dealer).

If you must do all or most of your jogging on the streets
and sidewalks, the major injury to watch is the "shin splint."

134

This is a pulling away of the muscles from the shinbone. If you begin to feel considerable pain in the shins after running regularly, discontinue jogging on hard surfaces for a while. An elastic bandage wrapped around the leg between the knee and the ankle will relieve some of the discomfort.

Don't run on your toes unless you're sprinting a short distance. If you run a long distance on your toes, you could end up with shin splints. Run with a flat-footed step, letting your heel touch the ground barely ahead of the rest of the foot.

Weather Problems

Don't use the weather as a reason not to jog. It's a good excuse for laziness, since you can find it either too hot, too cold, too rainy, too snowy, too slippery, or threatening to be any of the preceding. A friend used to say, "I'm going to start jogging as soon as the weather *breaks*." He could feel good about his intentions, but never had to worry about just when he would ever begin to jog. Waiting for the weather to break can keep you waiting a long time.

Some of the unique pleasures of jogging come when braving the cold, wind, snow, rain and hazardous terrain that inclement weather might bring. Some of the pleasure comes simply from being out there where the fainthearted will not go. But some of the pleasure also comes from the sense of control over your own body, mind, and even the threats of nature out there. It is the thrill of overcoming.

At the same time, we do not recommend that you jog during hail, sleet, or driving snowstorms. Jogging itself is not hindered much by these weather changes. But you can slip and fall easily, or you can be hit by an automobile out of control. Again, an important safety and health factor in inclement weather is proper warm-up. It is important to stretch the hamstring muscles (inside and back part of the upper leg) and the calf muscles (behind and below the knee). Stretching prevents muscle pulls. And in cold weather particularly, muscles become stiff (much like a rubber band becomes stiff and hard in the cold). Stretching will prevent undue strain.

Running involves more than just an occasional race. It involves training which makes a person into a finisher. The discipline of steady, continuous, and intense exercise is a means toward that end.

St. Paul knew that the exercise overload was important, not only for the body but also for the spirit. He said, "Like an athlete I punish my body, treating it roughly, training it to do what it should, not what it wants to. Otherwise I fear that after enlisting others for the race, I myself might be declared unfit and ordered to stand aside" (1 Cor. 9:27, TLB).

BIBLIOGRAPHY

American College of Sport Medicine. *Guidelines for Graded Exercise Testing and Exercise Prescription.* Philadelphia: Lea & Febiger, 1975.

Anderson, Bob. *Stretching.* Bolinas, CA: Shelter Publications, 1980.

Astrand, Per-Olaf & Rodahl, Kaare. *Textbook of Work Physiology,* New York: McGraw-Hill, 1970.

Baily, Covert. *Fit or Fat.* Boston: Houghton Mifflin, 1977.

Burkitt, D. P.,Walker, A. R., and Painter,N. X. "Dietary Fiber and Disease," *Journal of the American Medical Association,* Vol. 229, August 19, 1974.

Carter, Albert. *The Miracles of Rebound Exercise.* Edmonds, WA: The National Institute of Reboundology & Health, 1979.

Cooper, Kenneth H. *Aerobics.* New York: Evans & Company, 1968.

Cooper, Kenneth H. *The Aerobic Way.* New York: Bantam, 1978.

Diagram Group, The. *The Complete Encyclopedia of Exercise.* New York & London: Paddington Press, 1979.

Goldbeck, Nikki and David. *The Supermarket Handbook.* New York: The New American Library, 1976.

Johnson, Robert E. *U.S. Presidents Council on Physical Fitness and Sports Exercise and Weight Control.* Urbana, IL: University of Illinois Press, 1967.

La Lanne, Jack. *Slim and Trim Diet and Exercise Guide.* New York: Fawcett, n.d.

Layer, Susanne. "Diet Diseases." *W.S.U. Hilltop Magazine.* January, 1982.

Lune, David. *The Lean Machine.* Culver City, CA: Peace Press, 1980.

Merrill, Annabel L., and Watt, Bernice K. *Composition of Foods: Raw, Processed, Prepared.* U.S. Dept. of Agriculture, Consumer and Food Economics Institute, Agricultural Research Service, 1975.

Nutrition Search, Inc. *Nutrition Almanac.* New York: McGraw-Hill, 1975.

Pennington, Jean A.T., Church, Helen Nichols. *Food Values of Portions Commonly Used.* 13th Edition. New York: Harper & Row, 1980.

Rodale, J. I. *The Complete Book of Food and Nutrition.* Emmaus, PA: Rodale Books, 1972.

Rodale, J. I. *The Complete Book of Minerals for Health.* 4th Edition. Emmaus, PA: Rodale Books, 1976.

Thomas, Vaughan. *Science & Sport: How to Measure and Improve Athletic Performance.* Boston: Little, Brown, 1970.

White, James R. *Jump for Joy.* San Diego, CA; Goldfield Books, 1981.

Williams, Roger. *Biochemical Individuality.* Austin, TX; University of Texas Press, 1969.

Wilmore, Jack H. *Athletic Training & Physical Fitness: Physiological Principles and Practices of the Conditioning Process.* Boston: Allyn and Bacon, 1976.

Yudkin, John. *Sweet and Dangerous.* New York: Bantam Books, 1973.

ADDITIONAL READING MATERIAL

Exercise and Nutrition Books

Abrahamson, E.M. and Pezet, A.W. *Body, Mind and Sugar.* New York: Pyramid, 1951.

Airola, Paavo. *Hypoglycemia, A Better Approach.* Phoenix: Health Plus, 1977.

Brady, Jane. *Jane Brady's Nutrition Book.* New York: Norton, 1981.

Chapian, Marie. *Free To Be Thin.* Minneapolis: Bethany House Publishers, 1979.

Dufty, William. *Sugar Blues.* Radnor, PA: Chilton, 1975.

Gaines, Charles. *Staying Hard.* New York: Kenan Press, 1980.

Josephson, Elmer A. *God's Key to Health & Happiness.* Old Tappan, NJ: Revell, 1962.

Kilham, Christopher. *The Complete Shopper's Guide to Natural Foods.* Brookline, MA: Autumn Press, 1980.

Lappe, France Moore. *Diet for a Small Planet.* New York: Ballantine, 1971.

Lovett, C. S. *Help, Lord, the Devil Wants Me Fat.* Baldwin Park, CA: Personal Christianity, 1977.

Mindell, Earl. *Vitamin Bible.* New York: Warner Books, 1979.

Reuben, David. *The Save Your Life Diet.* New York: Ballantine, 1975.

Smith Lendon. *Foods for Healthy Kids.* New York: McGraw-Hill, 1981.

Cookbooks

Whyte, Karen Cross. *Complete Sprouting Cookbook.* San

Francisco: Troubador Press, 1973.

Ford, Marjorie Winn. *Deaf Smith Country Cookbook.* New York: Macmillan, 1973.

Geiskopt, Susan. *Putting It Up with Honey.* Ashland, OR: Quicksilver Productions, 1979.

Turnbull, Yvonne. *Living Cookbook.* Medford, OR: Omega Publications, 1981.

Magazines

Bestways, Box 2028, Carson City, NV. 89702.

Let's Live, 444 N. Larchmont Blvd., Los Angeles, CA. 90004.

Prevention, Rodale Press, 22 E. Minor St., Emmaus, PA. 18049.

Total Health, Trio Publications, 1800 N. Highland Ave., Ste. 720, Hollywood, CA. 90028.